Neuro Meds Made Easy

Callie Parker

Copyright

Copyright © 2025 by Callie Parker

All rights reserved.

No portion of this book may be reproduced in any form without written permission from the publisher or author, except as permitted by U.S. copyright law.

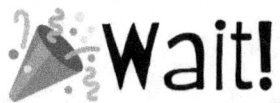

Wait!

Before You Dive In... Grab Your FREE Nursing Study Survival Kit!

Nursing school is no joke—that's why MadeEasy.Academy is committed to sending the ladder back down and rescuing those of you in the trenches!

Ready to study smarter, not harder? We've got exactly what you need.

Your FREE NCLEX in My Sleep Bundle Includes:

✅ Who's Dying First? The Prioritization Playbook: Because patient safety is kind of a big deal. 😅
✅ Flashcard Frenzy: Memorize or Die Trying: Pre-made Anki cards to save your sanity.
✅ WTF Does This Lab Value Mean? Cheat Sheet: No more second-guessing normal vs. "oh sh*t" levels.
✅ NCLEX Mnemonics That Stick (Like Tape on an IV Line): Memory hacks you'll actually remember.
✅ Med Math Without the Mental Breakdown: Because no one wants to commit a dosage error. 😬

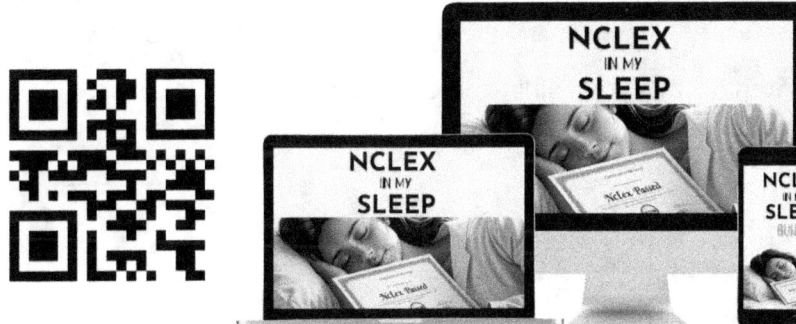

Head over to MadeEasy.Academy to grab your bundle. Let's turn nursing school stress into success!

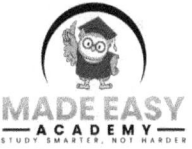

But that's not all...

🎁 BONUS 🎁

Your Bundle Includes an Exclusive 50% OFF Discount Code for your next course at Made Easy Academy
(Launching June 1!)

At <u>MadeEasy.Academy</u> we don't just simplify nursing—we transform it into an effortless, memorable study process.

For each topic, you'll follow our step by step success guide:

Step 1. Grab your cheat sheet: All key points, zero fluff.

Step 2. Read your mnemonic poem: Clever rhymes to make information stick.

Step 3. Take your fill-in-the-blank quiz: Test your recall without the overwhelm.

Step 4. Complete your NCLEX challenge: Realistic practice questions with clear rationales.

Step 5. Walk Into the NCLEX Like a Boss: Confident, prepared, and ready to pass.

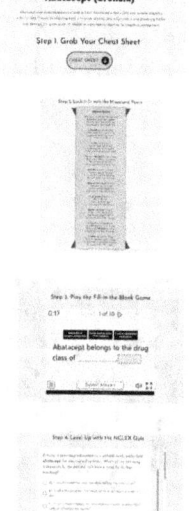
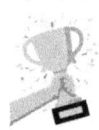

Right now, we're laser-focused on Pharmacology, but we'll soon expand into other crucial nursing topics! Have a topic you want us to cover next? Shoot us an email at hello@madeeasy.academy—we've got you!

Table of Contents

Made Easy: Why and How
Pharmacology Mind Maps
Pharmacology Mind Map Template
Neurotransmitters & Their Functions Chart
Pharmacology Mnemonics

Part I
Seizure & Antiepileptic Medications 1
   Brivaracetam (Briviact) 3
   Carbamazepine (Tegretol, Carbatrol) 4
   Cenobamate (Xcopri) 5
   Clobazam (Onfi) 6
   Clonazepam (Klonopin) 7
   Clonazepam ODT (Klonopin Wafer) 8
   Diazepam Rectal Gel (Diastat) 9
   Diazepam (Valium) 10
   Ethosuximide (Zarontin) 11
   Felbamate (Felbatol) 12
   Fenfluramine (Fintepla) 13
   Gabapentin (Neurontin) 14
   Gabapentin Enacarbil (Horizant) 15
   Lamotrigine (Lamictal) 16
   Lacosamide (Vimpat) 17
   Levetiracetam (Keppra) 18
   Lorazepam IV (Ativan) 19
   Oxcarbazepine (Trileptal) 20
   Perampanel (Fycompa) 21
   Phenobarbital (Luminal) 22
   Phenytoin (Dilantin) 23
   Pregabalin (Lyrica) 24
   Primidone (Mysoline) 25
   Propranolol (Inderal) 26
   Rufinamide (Banzel) 27
   Topiramate (Topamax) 28
   Valproic Acid (Depakote) 29
   Vigabatrin (Sabril) 30
   Zonisamide (Zonegran) 31

Part II
Parkinson's & Movement Disorders ... 33
- Amantadine (Symmetrel, Gocovri) ... 35
- Apomorphine (Apokyn) ... 36
- Apomorphine Sublingual (Kynmobi) ... 37
- Benztropine (Cogentin) ... 38
- Carbidopa/Levodopa (Sinemet) ... 39
- Entacapone (Comtan) ... 40
- Pramipexole (Mirapex) ... 41
- Rasagiline (Azilect) ... 42
- Ropinirole (Requip) ... 43
- Ropinirole ER (Requip XL) ... 44
- Rotigotine (Neupro) ... 45
- Safinamide (Xadago) ... 46
- Selegiline (Eldepryl, Zelapar) ... 47
- Selegiline Patch (Emsam) ... 48
- Tolcapone (Tasmar) ... 49
- Trihexyphenidyl (Artane) ... 50
- Istradefylline (Nourianz) ... 51

Part III
Multiple Sclerosis & Autoimmune Neuro Meds ... 52
- Alemtuzumab (Lemtrada) ... 54
- Cladribine (Mavenclad) ... 55
- Dimethyl Fumarate (Tecfidera) ... 56
- Fingolimod (Gilenya) ... 57
- Glatiramer Acetate (Copaxone) ... 58
- Interferon Beta-1a (Avonex, Rebif) ... 59
- Interferon Beta-1b (Betaseron) ... 60
- Mitoxantrone (Novantrone) ... 61
- Natalizumab (Tysabri) ... 62
- Ocrelizumab (Ocrevus) ... 63
- Ofatumumab (Kesimpta) ... 64
- Ozanimod (Zeposia) ... 65
- Peginterferon Beta-1a (Plegridy) ... 66
- Ponesimod (Ponvory) ... 67
- Siponimod (Mayzent) ... 68
- Teriflunomide (Aubagio) ... 69

Part IV
Migraine & CGRP Antagonists ... 70
- Almotriptan (Axert) ... 72
- Atogepant (Qulipta) ... 73
- Dihydroergotamine (Migranal) ... 74
- Eletriptan (Relpax) ... 75

Eptinezumab (Vyepti)...76
Erenumab (Aimovig)..77
Fremanezumab (Ajovy)...78
Frovatriptan (Frova)..79
Galcanezumab (Emgality)..80
Lasmiditan (Reyvow)..81
Naratriptan (Amerge)..82
Rizatriptan (Maxalt)..83
Rimegepant (Nurtec ODT)...84
Sumatriptan (Imitrex)...85
Ubrogepant (Ubrelvy)..86
Zolmitriptan (Zomig)..87
Zavegepant (Zavzpret)..88

Part V
Alzheimer's, Dementia & Cognitive Decline........................90
Donepezil (Aricept)..92
Galantamine (Razadyne, Razadyne ER)............................93
Memantine (Namenda)...94
Methylphenidate Patch (Daytrana)....................................95
Rivastigmine (Exelon)..96

Part VI
Sleep, Sedatives & Restless Legs..98
Butalbital/Acetaminophen/Caffeine (Fioricet)...............100
Eszopiclone (Lunesta)...101
Lorazepam (Ativan)...102
Midazolam (Nayzilam)..103
Temazepam (Restoril)...104
Suvorexant (Belsomra)...105
Solriamfetol (Sunosi)..106
Hydroxyzine (Vistaril)..107
Zolpidem (Ambien)..108

Part VII
ADHD, Stimulants & Wakefulness...110
Armodafinil (Nuvigil)..112
Atomoxetine (Strattera)...113
Dexedrine (Dextroamphetamine Sulfate)......................114
Solriamfetol (Sunosi)..115
Dexmethylphenidate (Focalin)...116
Dextroamphetamine/Amphetamine (Adderall)..........117
Guanfacine (Intuniv)...118
Lisdexamfetamine (Vyvanse)..119

Methylphenidate (Ritalin, Concerta) 120
Modafinil (Provigil) 121

Part VIII
Depression, Anxiety & Mood Stabilizers **122**
Amitriptyline (Elavil) 123
Armodafinil (Nuvigil) 124
Buspirone (Buspar) 125
Selegiline (Eldepryl, Zelapar) 126
Selegiline Patch (Emsam) 127
Duloxetine (Cymbalta) 128
Milnacipran (Savella) 129
Nortriptyline (Pamelor) 130
Pimavanserin (Nuplazid) 131

Part IX
Muscle Relaxants, Motion & Myasthenia **132**
Baclofen (Lioresal) 134
Dantrolene (Dantrium) 135
Edrophonium (Tensilon) 136
Efgartigimod (Vyvgart) 137
Meclizine (Antivert) 138
Tizanidine (Zanaflex) 139
Pyridostigmine (Mestinon) 140
Scopolamine Patch (Transderm Scop) 141
Toviaz (Fesoterodine) 142

Part X
Miscellaneous Neurology **144**
Acetazolamide (Diamox) 146
Amifampridine (Firdapse) 147
Cannabidiol (Epidiolex) 148
Dalfampridine (Ampyra) 149
Deutetrabenazine (Austedo) 150
Dextromethorphan/Quinidine (Nuedexta) 151
Droxidopa (Northera) 152
Edaravone (Radicava) 153
Lidocaine Patch (Lidoderm) 154
Riluzole (Rilutek) 155
Risdiplam (Evrysdi) 156
Sodium Oxybate (Xyrem) 157
Tetrabenazine (Xenazine) 158
Valbenazine (Ingrezza) 159

WHY Made Easy Works

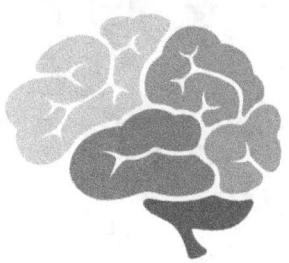

Backed by Brain Science

Let's face it — nursing school can feel like trying to drink from a firehose. Between the jargon, the never-ending lists, and the sheer volume of information, it's easy to feel overwhelmed. That's exactly why the Made Easy series was born: to make the hard stuff stick without frying your brain. And while it might look fun and playful on the outside (hello, rhymes!), it's all built on rock-solid research from the nerdy world of educational psychology.

1. COGNITIVE LOAD THEORY

First up: Cognitive Load Theory. Fancy name, simple idea — your brain can only handle so much at once. When materials are too dense or packed with fluff, your working memory taps out. Educational psychologist John Sweller figured this out, and we took notes. That's why our poems give you the essentials only, in small, memorable doses. Less clutter, more clarity. (Sweller, 1988; Clark et al., 2006)

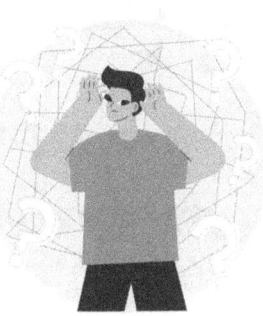

2. DUAL CODING THEORY

Then there's Dual Coding Theory, brought to us by Allan Paivio. He discovered that we remember things better when we learn them through both words and visuals. Our poems lean into this by using rhyme and rhythm to boost verbal memory — and bolded key terms, color coding, and clean formatting to give your visual brain a treat. Two paths to your brain = double the retention. (Paivio, 1986; Mayer, 2009)

3. ADVANCE ORGANIZERS

Psychologist David Ausubel believed that when we know how new info fits into what we already know, we learn faster. That's the beauty of our repeatable poem structure. Once you get the hang of the format, your brain relaxes – and focuses on what actually matters: the content. Think of it like a familiar playlist for your mind. (Ausubel, 1960)

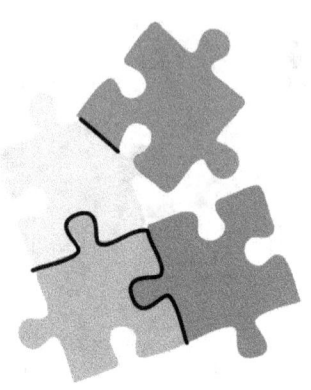

4. MICROLEARNING

Our poems are also bite-sized by design, and that's no accident. Welcome to the world of microlearning – the idea that small, focused learning units are easier to digest and retain. This is a game-changer for busy, burnt-out students. Instead of cramming for hours, you can study just one medication, one skill, or one critical concept at a time. Snack-sized studying with full-course impact. (Hug, 2005; van den Berg & van den Berg, 2021)

5. SPACED REPETITION & RETRIEVAL PRACTICE

Last but definitely not least: spaced repetition and retrieval practice. These two learning powerhouses have proven time and again that the more often you recall information over time, the longer you'll remember it. Our poems are made for this. Easy to reread, perfect for flashcards, and fun enough to come back to (yes, we admitted it). Rinse and repeat – and retain. (Dunlosky et al., 2013)

So, yes – this method might look different than your typical textbook grind. That's the point. It's effective on purpose. Because learning tough topics shouldn't feel impossible. It should feel doable. Even a little fun. And with Made Easy, it totally is.

Read it. Rhyme it. Remember it.

That's the Made Easy Method—a simple but powerful approach to mastering complex nursing material.

ONE — START WITH THE BIG PICTURE

Before diving into individual medications, review the Mind Maps (via QR code). These quick-reference visuals give you the foundational understanding needed for any medication.

Included mind maps:
- The Life of a Drug in the Body (pharmacokinetics)
- Drug Classifications
- Common Side Effect Categories
- High-Risk Medication Categories
- Drug Schedules (I-V)
- Therapeutic Index & Drug Monitoring
- Common Drug Interactions
- Ways to Memorize Meds

These are perfect for test prep, concept review, and connecting the dots across drug types.

USE THE MEMORY TRICKS & MNEMONICS — TWO

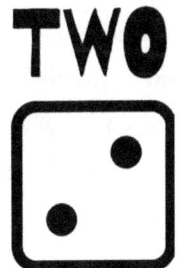

We've included 2 pages of mnemonic "cards" — visual reminders of popular phrases and acronyms students actually use (and remember!).

Cut them out, hang them up, or snap a pic to review on the go.

THREE 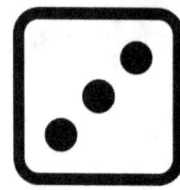 STUDY WITH PURPOSE

Don't just read — actively study.

As you go through each medication, we encourage you to highlight or underline using this color-coded system to instantly recognize what's what:

- ▪ Drug Classification & Names
- ▪ Mechanism of Action
- ▪ Indications
- ▪ Side Effects & Adverse Reactions
- ▪ Nursing Considerations
- Monitoring Requirements
- ▪ Patient & Caregiver Teaching Points
- ● Black Box Warnings
- Pediatric Considerations
- ● Drug Interactions

(Pro Tip: You don't need 10 highlighters — just make a little color key and underline or box with gel pens or colored pencils!)

COMPLETE THE MIND MAP   FOUR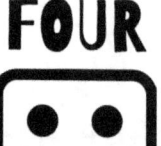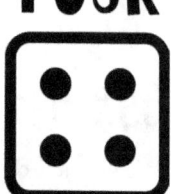

Once you've highlighted, it's time to organize what you've learned. Use the Medication Mind Map Template in the back of the book to visually break down the drug:

- Class, MOA, Indications
- Side effects, warnings, teaching points
- Your favorite memory trick or mnemonic

This helps you actually process and remember what you just studied — way better than passive reading.

FIVE

TEST WHAT YOU KNOW

After each section, you'll find a QR code that takes you straight to a short NCLEX-style quiz hosted in Google Forms. These aren't just random practice questions – they're carefully crafted to test the most important takeaways from what you just read. But the real magic? <u>The rationales.</u> Whether you get the answer right or wrong, the quiz walks you through the why. Understanding the reasoning behind each answer helps you think like a nurse, not just a test-taker.

It's not about memorizing – it's about making connections, strengthening critical thinking, and applying your knowledge in real clinical scenarios. So take your time, review the rationales, and let them guide you from confusion to clarity.

So don't just read these pages—
interact with them.

📖 **Read it.** 🎵 **Rhyme it.** 🧠 **Remember it.**

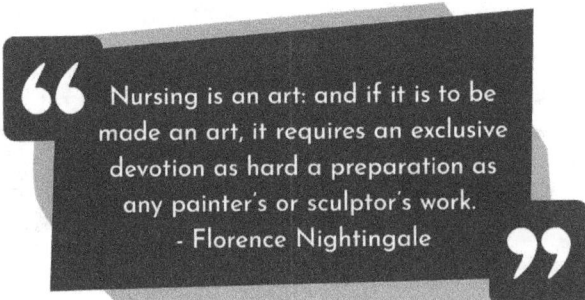

> Nursing is an art: and if it is to be made an art, it requires an exclusive devotion as hard a preparation as any painter's or sculptor's work.
> - Florence Nightingale

PHARMACOLOGY MIND MAPS

COMMON DRUG INTERACTIONS

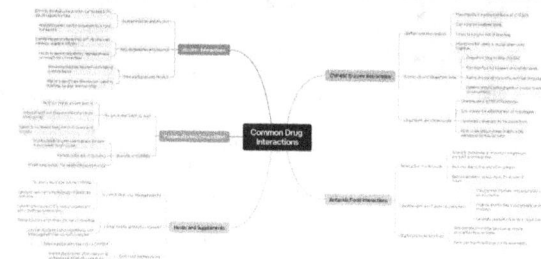

THE LIFE OF A DRUG IN THE BODY

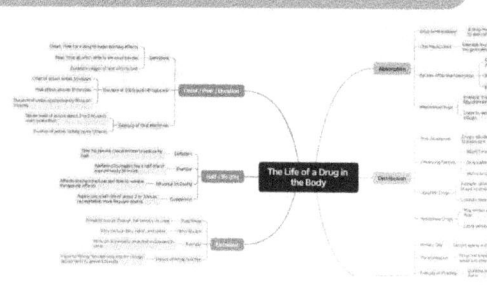

DRUG CLASSIFICATIONS

HIGH-RISK MEDICATION CATEGORIES

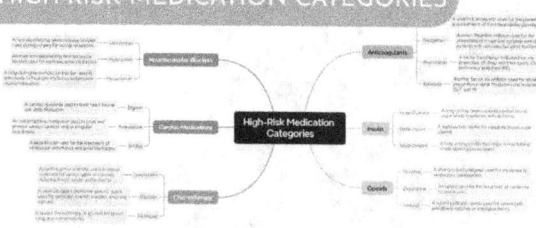

DRUG SCHEDULES

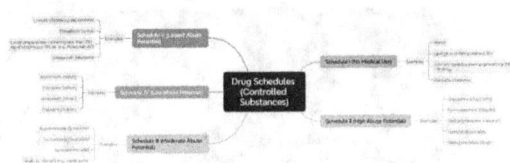

THERAPEUTIC INDEX & DRUG MONITORING

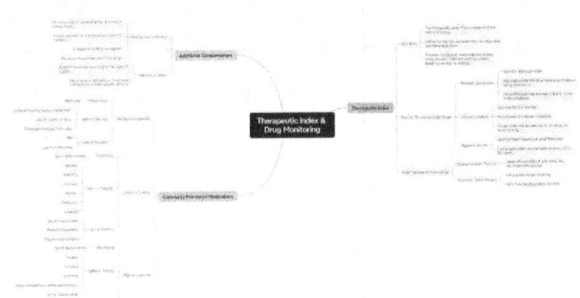

COMMON DRUG INTERACTIONS

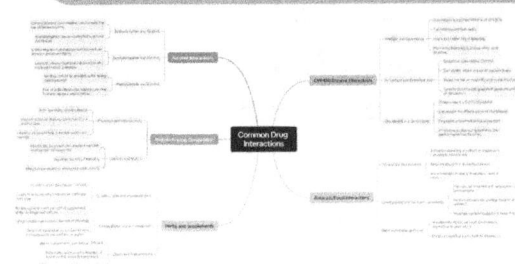

WAYS TO MEMORIZE MEDICATIONS

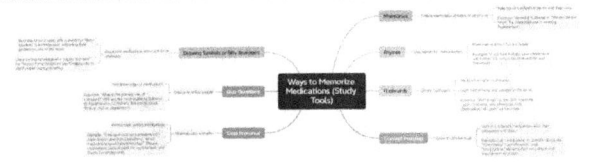

NEUROTRANSMITTERS & THEIR FUNCTIONS

Neurotransmitter	Main Function	If Decreased	If Increased	Associated Meds
Dopamine	Pleasure, motivation, motor control	Parkinson's, depression	Schizophrenia, psychosis	Antipsychotics, Levodopa, Bupropion
Serotonin	Mood, sleep, appetite	Depression, anxiety	Serotonin syndrome	SSRIs, SNRIs, Triptans
Norepinephrine	Fight/flight, focus, arousal	Depression, hypotension	Anxiety, hypertension	SNRIs, MAOIs, Beta-blockers
GABA	Calming, inhibits CNS	Anxiety, seizures	Sedation	Benzos, barbiturates, Gabapentin
Glutamate	Learning, memory, excitatory signal	Poor cognition	Seizures, neurotoxicity	NMDA antagonists (Memantine)
Acetylcholine	Memory, learning, muscle control	Alzheimer's, myasthenia	Cholinergic crisis	Donepezil, Rivastigmine, Anticholinergics

Pharm Mnemonics

SLUDGE
CHOLINERGIC EFFECTS

Salivation, **L**acrimation, **U**rination, **D**iaphoresis, **G**I upset, **E**mesis

Seen in cholinergic overdose or organophosphate poisoning.

ANTICHOLINERGIC
Can't Pee, See, Spit, or Poop

Blurred vision, Urinary retention, Dry mouth, Constipation

Helps recall the hallmark side effects of anticholinergic medications.

NAMES OF INSULINS - L.A.N.D.

Lantus = Long-acting
Apidra = Rapid-acting
Novolog = Rapid-acting
Detemir = Long-acting

BETA-BLOCKERS

"**LOL** Makes the Heart Rate Slow"

All beta-blockers end in "-lol." They decrease heart rate and blood pressure by blocking beta-adrenergic receptors.

ACE INHIBITORS

"-**PRIL** Puts the Pressure Down"

Pressure Reduced In Large vessels. They lower blood pressure by preventing angiotensin II formation.

CALCIUM CHANNEL BLOCKERS

"**V**ery **N**ice **D**rugs"
Verapamil, **N**ifedipine, **D**iltiazem

These drugs dilate blood vessels and slow the heart rate, reducing workload on the heart.

DIURETICS

"**DIM** the Fluid Volume"

Diuretics, **I**ncrease, **M**icturition (urination)

Loop diuretics (e.g., furosemide) or thiazides (e.g., hydrochlorothiazide) help reduce fluid volume, easing edema or hypertension.

ANTICOAGULANTS

"Heparin Works **FAST**, Coumadin **LASTS**"

Heparin is for acute management; Warfarin for long-term prevention. Always monitor lab values (PTT for heparin, PT/INR for warfarin).

ANTIBIOTICS (PENICILLINS & CEPHALOSPORINS)

"Cross Allergy Alerts"

All beta-blockers end in "-lol." They decrease heart rate and blood pressure by blocking beta-adrenergic receptors.

LIDOCAINE TOXICITY

"**SAMS**"
Slurred speech, **A**ltered central nervous system, **M**uscle twitching, **S**eizures

Recognize signs of lidocaine toxicity.

MEDICATION ADMINISTRATION CHECKLIST

"**TRAMP**"

Time, **R**oute, **A**mount, **M**edication, **P**atient

Ensure the five rights of medication administration.

EMERGENCY DRUGS TO "**LEAN**" ON

Lidocaine, **E**pinephrine, **A**tropine, **N**aloxone

Common emergency medications administered via endotracheal tube.

Pharm Mnemonics

VENTRICULAR ARRHYTHMIAS
"PALS"
Procainamide, Amiodarone, Lidocaine, Sotalol

Medications used to treat ventricular arrhythmias.

ATRIAL ARRHYTHMIAS
"ABCDE"
Anticoagulants, Beta blockers, Calcium channel blockers, Digoxin, Electrocardioversion

Treatment options for atrial arrhythmias.

MORPHINE SIDE EFFECTS
"MORPHINE"
Miosis, Out of it (sedation), Respiratory depression, Pneumonia (aspiration), Hypotension, Infrequency (constipation, urinary retention), Nausea, Emesis

PARKINSON'S MEDICATIONS
"ALBM"
Amantadine, Levodopa, Bromocriptine, MAO-B inhibitors

Drugs commonly used to manage Parkinson's disease.

THIAZIDES INDICATIONS
"CHIC"
Congestive heart failure, Hypertension, Insipidus (diabetes insipidus), Calcium calculi (kidney stones)

Primary uses for thiazide diuretics.

BRADYCARDIA & HYPOTENSION
"IDEA"
Isoproterenol, Dopamine, Epinephrine, Atropine sulfate

Medications used to manage bradycardia and hypotension.

STEROID SIDE EFFECTS
"6 S's"
Sugar - hyperglycemia, Soggy bones - osteoporosis, Sick - decreased immunity, Sad - depression, Salt - water and salt retention, Sex - decreased libido

LOOP DIURETIC EFFECTS
"LOOP"
Lose sodium, Ototoxicity, Orthostatic hypotension, Potassium loss

Highlights the primary effects and risks of loop diuretics.

ACE INHIBITOR SIDE EFFECTS
"CAPTOPRIL"
Cough, Angioedema, Proteinuria, Taste changes, Orthostatic hypotension, Pregnancy contraindication, Rash, Increased renin, Lower angiotensin II

BETA-BLOCKER CONTRAINDICATIONS
"ABCDE"
Asthma, Block (heart block), COPD, Diabetes mellitus, Electrolyte (hyperkalemia)

Highlights conditions where beta-blockers should be used cautiously or avoided.

GYNECOMASTIA
"DISCO"
Digitalis, Isoniazid, Spironolactone, Cimetidine, Oestrogens

Identifies medications known to cause gynecomastia as a side effect.

TOXICOLOGICAL SEIZURES
"OTIS CAMPBELL"
Organophosphates, Tricyclic antidepressants, Isoniazid, Insulin, Sympathomimetics, Camphor, Cocaine, Amphetamines, Methylxanthines, PCP, Propoxyphene, Phenol, Propranolol, Benzodiazepine withdrawal, Botanicals, Ethanol withdrawal, Lithium, Lidocaine, Lindane, Lead

Part I
Seizure & Antiepileptic Medications

BRIVARACETAM (BRIVIACT)
Antiepileptic / Anticonvulsant

For **seizure storms** that strike at will,
Brivaracetam helps things stay still.
It binds to **SV2A**, fast and sleek,
To calm the brain when signals peak.
A **partial-onset seizure** aid,
In **adults and kids**, it makes the grade.
It slows the sparks, brings quiet back,
By modulating synaptic track.

Side effects can cloud the day:
Drowsiness, **dizziness** in the way.
Fatigue, **nausea**, **mood swings** too,
And sometimes **anger** breaking through.
There's risk of **suicidal thoughts**,
So screen for mental warning spots.
And though it's rare, **hypersensitivity**
Can bring a rash or worse activity.

Monitor for mood decline,
Watch **coordination** over time.
Check for **infection**—it may show,
As **neutrophils** can run too low.
Teach patients not to stop too fast—
Withdrawal seizures might come back fast.
Let them know to **watch for mood**,
And **report aggression** if it intrudes.

No **black box warning**, but still alert
To **psychiatric shifts** that can hurt.
Avoid with heavy **alcohol sways**,
It enhances drowsiness and haze.
Interactions? Not too many—
But **rifampin** can make levels skinny.
And though it's cousin to **levetiracetam**,
It's **more selective** in the synaptic jam.

So **Brivaracetam**, with its grace,
Brings seizure calm to a hectic place.
Used with care, it holds the line—
A steady shield for the neural spine.

CARBAMAZEPINE (TEGRETOL, CARBATROL)
Anticonvulsant / Mood Stabilizer

When **neurons misfire**, sparks run wild,
Carbamazepine keeps things mild.
It **blocks sodium channels** deep,
To help those firing patterns sleep.
Used for **partial seizures**, and **tonic-clonic**,
And in **bipolar** swings that get demonic.
Also tames **trigeminal nerve pain**,
When electric shocks strike face and brain.
But tread with care—**side effects** are wide:
Dizziness, drowsiness, mood may slide.
Ataxia, nausea, blurry view,
Leukopenia may come through.
Serious risks? Let's make them known:
SJS, TEN, where skin is blown.
More common in **Asian descent**,
If **HLA-B*1502** is present—test before it's sent.
Also **aplastic anemia**, a rare concern,
And **agranulocytosis**—watch and learn.
So **CBCs** are key to check,
And any sign of fever—inspect!
Monitor: CBCs, LFTs, and drug levels,
Especially when seizure threshold revels.
It's also an **auto-inducer**, mind—
It speeds up its own clearance over time.
Teach patients: **don't crush XR**,
And take with **food** to go far.

Avoid **grapefruit juice**—it interferes,
And causes levels to shift gears.
Black box warnings loud and clear:
Blood dyscrasias and **skin rashes** near.
And watch for **suicide warning signs**,
As mood may dip between the lines.
Drug interactions? A hefty list:
It lowers levels of many missed.
Warfarin, OCPs, and more can fade—
So double-check the drugs they've made.
So **Carbamazepine**, strong and sure,
Brings seizures and wild moods a cure.
But guide its use with watchful eyes,
To keep the brain safe, sharp, and wise.

CENOBAMATE (XCOPRI)
Antiepileptic / Anticonvulsant

When **partial seizures** crash the brain,
And other meds don't dull the strain,
Cenobamate comes on strong—
To calm the currents that go wrong.
It **blocks sodium channels**, sleek,
And **modulates GABA** to make things meek.
By quieting the neural storm,
It brings a more **controlled brain form**.

Approved for **adults with focal flare**,
When seizures strike from here to there.
Not first in line—but when things fail,
Xcopri helps to **tip the scale**.
Side effects you'll need to note:
Drowsiness, dizziness, fatigue's big coat.
Also **headache, double sight**,
And **coordination** not quite right.

Some face **serious risks** in kind:
DRESS syndrome—keep that in mind.
A rash with **fever, organ pain**—
Could be fatal, so explain.
Start **low and slow**, that's the rule,
Titrate weekly, keep it cool.
Monitor sodium, ECG too—
QT shortening can sneak through.

Watch for **mental health decline**,
And check for **suicidal sign**.
Avoid abrupt stops—taper instead,
Or seizures might come back full spread.

Teach patients: **no alcohol**,
And take at night to avoid the sprawl.
May take weeks to feel the best—
So stick with it, then assess.

No **black box warning** yet, it's true,
But rare reactions may accrue.
Drug interactions? Yes, a pile—
It changes levels with some style.
Phenytoin, phenobarb, and more—
And may reduce birth control's score.
Also, **CYP inhibitors** may raise its might,
So monitor labs to get it right.

So **Cenobamate**, new and strong,
Can help when seizures last too long.
With patient care and slow build pace,
It brings back calm—and clearer space.

CLOBAZAM (ONFI)
Benzodiazepine / Antiepileptic

When **seizures flare** in clustered waves,
And other meds no longer save,
Clobazam steps in with care—
To calm the storm with **benzo flair**.
It's a **benzodiazepine**, you see,
But different in its **structure tree**.
Less sedating than the rest,
Yet still it helps the brain find rest.

Used for **Lennox-Gastaut** in kids and grown,
Where seizure types are widely sown.
Also used **off-label** wide—
For panic, spasms, and the like.
It **boosts GABA** at its core,
Opening channels to calm the roar.
Inhibits neurons gone too loud,
And helps the brain feel less unbowed.

Side effects include the norm:
Drowsiness, lethargy, not top form.
Aggression, irritability, or **mood decline**,
Ataxia, drooling, across the line.
Serious risks include **withdrawal**,
And **respiratory depression** call.
Especially with **opioids** or **sedatives** near,
This benzo's effects can interfere.

Monitor for changes in tone,
Mood, **sleep**, or if seizures are still shown.
Also check for **drug tolerance** climb—
It can lose effect over time.
Teach patients: Don't just **stop or quit**,
Taper slowly, bit by bit.
Caution with **alcohol** or **sleepy meds**,
And **no machinery** until clear heads.

Black box warning? Yes, a bold one:
For **concurrent opioid use**, it's no fun.
It raises risk for **coma, breath**,
And may even lead to **sudden death**.
Drug interactions include CYP,
3A4 and **2C19** may flip.
Inhibitors can raise its level high,
So check those scripts before they fly.

So **Clobazam**, a steady light,
Brings seizure calm without full night.
A benzo built for longer stay—
But only safe the careful way.

CLONAZEPAM (KLONOPIN)
Benzodiazepine / Antiepileptic / Anxiolytic

When **nerves misfire** or **panic creeps**,
Clonazepam brings calming sleeps.
It's a **benzodiazepine** that slows
The wildest of neuronal flows.
It **boosts GABA**'s soothing power,
To ease the storm in anxious hour.
Used for **seizures, panic, restless legs**,
And sometimes when the whole brain begs.
It treats **Lennox-Gastaut** and more,
With **myoclonic jerks** or **tonic-clonic war**.
Also for **panic disorders**, grim,
And **off-label uses** on a whim.
Side effects include the known:
Drowsiness, dizziness, slowed-down tone.
Ataxia, slurred speech, and sometimes fear,
Behavioral shifts may soon appear.
Long-term use may start to fade,
As **tolerance** and **dependence** get made.
And withdrawal—**seizures, tremors, dread**,
If stopped too fast—**taper instead**.
Monitor for sedation signs,
And worsening of anxious minds.
Respiratory status if you dare
To combine with **opioids**—handle with care.
Teach patients: **don't crush or chew**,
Take it **as prescribed** and true.
Warn of **falls, no alcohol**, and if mood
Turns dark or odd—report that, too.
Black box warning—yes, it's clear:
With **opioids**, life-threatening risks appear.
Coma, death, or **breathing slow**,
Especially in the **elderly flow**.
Drug interactions? Quite a few—
With **CNS depressants**, and **valproate**, too.
Also **azole antifungals** raise the ride,
And may push levels to the side.
So **Clonazepam**, long in fame,
Can calm the brain and tame the flame.
But use with caution, slow and wise,
To keep the risk from ever rise.

CLONAZEPAM ODT (KLONOPIN WAFER)

Seizure & Sedative - Sublingual Benzodiazepine

A **benzo wafer**, quick to take, It melts with ease — no need to shake. For **seizures**, **panic**, or **distress**, It calms the nerves and soothes the stress.
It binds to **GABA-A** receptor site, Enhancing **calm**, suppressing **fright**. By slowing **CNS signals** down, It quells the **twitch**, the **fear**, the **frown**.
The **ODT** is meant to melt, **Sublingual** dosing safely dealt. For patients who can't **swallow well**, This form ensures that care goes swell.
It's used for **seizure prophylaxis**, Or **acute spikes**, like **spastic axis**. Also helpful when **fear's too strong**, Or **panic attacks** are lasting too long.
Its **onset's quick, effects profound**, Within an hour it's working round.
Duration varies — **long half-life**, So **steady state** avoids much strife.
Side effects include **sedation**, **Ataxia** and **concentration frustration**. Watch for **dizziness** or **slurred tone**, Especially if the patient's prone.
Caution when used with **other meds**, Especially those that **knock in beds**. Avoid with **alcohol** and **sleep pills**, Combo use may lead to chills.
Withdrawal risk is high and real, So **taper slow** — that's part of the deal. From **shaking limbs** to **rapid heart**, Benzo withdrawal plays no part.
In **pregnancy**, there's some concern, **Malformations** — so rethink and learn. In **lactation**, the risk is real, **Monitor baby** with every meal.
Controlled as Schedule Number Four, **Addiction risk** you can't ignore. Use **short-term** when possible, **Long-term use** is tossable.
Monitor mood and **suicide risk**, Though rare, it still can coexist. And check for **liver** working fine, Before you give this classic line.
So when you choose this **ODT**, Remember **bioavailability**. It's **quick**, it's **clean**, and doesn't choke, But treat it with respect — no joke.

DIAZEPAM RECTAL GEL (DIASTAT)

Emergency Benzodiazepine – Status Epilepticus

A **rescue med**, for when it's dire,
To stop the brain from **rapid fire**.
Rectal gel in **pre-filled tubes**, For seizing patients — no time to lose.
A **benzodiazepine** by class, It helps those **seizure storms** to pass. It binds to **GABA**, slows the flow, So **overstimulation** won't grow.
Used when **status** takes its hold, And **IV access** can't unfold. In **homes**, in **schools**, or **EMS**, This med can quickly de-stress.
It's **not for daily seizure care**, But **emergencies** that strip you bare. When **two or more seizures** hit, And don't stop — this **gel's a fit**.
Onset is fast, within **five to ten**, Though **watch for breathing issues** then. **Respiratory depression**'s real — So **monitor the breath** and feel.
Sedation, slurred speech, dizzy ways, Might linger on for hours or days. **Hypotension** may occur, And **loss of balance** might transfer.
The **dose** is based on **weight and age**, So fill out clearly on the page. Prescribed with **lock**, it won't dispense, Until the **dose makes common sense**.
Administer while on their side, Insert with **lube**, and don't be shy. Hold the **cheeks** for three full ticks, Then **remove** and wait — no tricks.
Stay close for **fifteen minutes flat**, If they don't wake, it's time to act. Call the team, prepare to ride, Further help must now decide.
It's **Schedule IV**, and **stored with care**, No **fridge** is needed anywhere. **Teach the family** when to give, So the patient has a chance to live.
Don't give it **twice** without a guide, Or mix with meds that **tranquilize**. **One dose**, then seek **medical aid**, So future seizures can be weighed. Respect the gel and what it's for — It opens up a **rescue door**. And when IV lines just can't begin, **Diastat** is the win within.

DIAZEPAM (VALIUM)

Benzodiazepine / Antianxiety / Anticonvulsant / Muscle Relaxant

When **nerves are tense** or **muscles shake**,
And sleep won't come for calmness' sake,
Diazepam—the **Valium** name—
Helps bring the brain back in the game.
A **benzodiazepine** so smooth,
It **amplifies GABA** to help soothe.
That **chloride flood** calms neurons down,
And takes away the anxious frown.
Used for **anxiety**, **seizures**, too,
And **muscle spasms** out of the blue.
Also for **alcohol withdrawal's** bite,
And **status epilepticus** at night.
Side effects? A sleepy slide:
Drowsiness, fatigue, and brain fog wide.
Ataxia, slurred speech, blurred-out gaze,
And **confusion** in the older phase.
Respiratory depression risk
Goes up with **opioids**, that mix is brisk.
Add **tolerance, dependence, withdrawal pain**,
If stopped too fast—it's not so plain.
Monitor sedation, breathing slow,
And **fall risk**, especially in those
Who are **elderly**, frail, or new
To meds that make the CNS stew.
Teach patients: don't **drink with this**,
And don't just stop—it's not hit or miss.
Use **short-term**, not as a crutch,
Long-term risks? There's more than much.
Black box warning? Yes, it's here:
Opioid combos—danger clear.
May cause **coma**, **death**, or breath to fade,
So use with caution, don't be swayed.
Drug interactions? A broad terrain—
With **CNS depressants**, it hits the brain.
And **CYP3A4 inhibitors**, too,
May **raise the levels** more than due.
So **Diazepam**, though tried and true,
Needs careful hands to guide it through.
It soothes, relaxes, calms the tide—
But only when it's safely prescribed.

ETHOSUXIMIDE (ZARONTIN)

Antiepileptic / Succinimide Class - Absence Seizure Agent

When **blank stares** steal time away,
And kids just **zone out** mid-school day,
Ethosuximide leads the charge,
To keep those **absence seizures** small, not large.
It **blocks calcium channels**—T-type, low,
To stop the **thalamus' rhythmic glow**.
That tiny spark that loops too long
Is quieted so brains stay strong.
Used for **absence seizures**, it's first in line—
For **petit mal** types, it works just fine.
Not for tonic, not for clonic,
It's specific—and iconic.
Side effects are mostly mild,
But monitor each **epileptic child**.
GI upset, like **cramps** and **pain**,
Weight loss, **hiccups**, might remain.
Drowsiness, dizziness, headache, too,
And **behavioral changes** coming through.
In rare cases, something more—
SJS, leukopenia, knocking at the door.
Monitor CBC and LFT,
Especially for those on it long-term, you see.
And check for rash or fever climb—
Could signal trouble just in time.
Teach families it may take a while
For full effects to show and smile.
Doses start low, then rise with care,
And should be taken same time, fair.
No black box warning, but stay aware—
Of serious reactions, though they're rare.
And if **suicidal thoughts** are seen,
Refer, report, and intervene.
Drug interactions? A modest spread—
Watch with **valproate, phenytoin** tread.
Levels can shift, so check and tweak,
Especially if control gets weak.
So **Zarontin**, simple, steady, small,
Can stop the seizures' silent call.
A focused med for minds that drift—
To bring young brains a subtle lift.

FELBAMATE (FELBATOL)
Antiepileptic - Reserved Use Only

Felbamate, a seizure tool, Reserved for when the risks still rule. Used when others fail to do, But **high-risk effects** must be in view.

It treats **Lennox-Gastaut** and more, When daily seizures flood the floor. It blocks **NMDA**, calms the brain, And modulates the **sodium** train.

It enhances **GABA-A** too, To slow the spikes that cut right through. A complex mech, but here's the gist: It quiets nerves with every twist. Yet while it works, the dangers bite, Its use is rare and always tight.

Aplastic anemia may arise— A sudden loss of blood cell ties. And worse, it may **destroy the liver**, A risk that makes most doctors shiver. So check **LFTs** before you start, And warn the patient from the heart.

It's only used with **informed consent**, And after safer drugs are spent. Each patient signs before they take, A risk form for their safety's sake.

Headache, **dizzy**, **weight loss** too, And **insomnia** can come through. But all these pale when you compare, To liver loss and marrow scare.

It may **raise phenytoin** levels fast, So monitor drugs that tend to last. Interactions? Yes, there's more— Watch **carbamazepine** to the core.

Dosing starts out fairly slow, Then titrate up, but never go Without checking labs on cue— This med needs **labs and oversight** too.

It's **not first-line**, that's understood, But sometimes, risks are weighed for good. For seizure types that don't give rest, This med is used when all else stressed.

So **Felbamate**, though rare in play, Deserves respect in every way. It's not the star—but in a storm, It may just help a brain transform.

FENFLURAMINE (FINTEPLA)

Antiepileptic / Serotonin Releaser / Seizure Control Agent

When **seizures strike in endless tide**,
And **Dravet syndrome** won't subside,
Fenfluramine steps up the fight,
To **calm the storm** and bring in light.
It's not your typical seizure med—
It works with **serotonin** instead.
By boosting levels in the brain,
It **modulates excitatory strain**.

Also touches **sigma-1**,
To help reduce those seizures' run.
It's used when others fail to tame
The **frequent seizures** that inflame.
Side effects? Yes, be alert:
Fatigue, diarrhea, sleep disturb hurt.
Decreased appetite, weight loss, too,
And **fevers, infections** may come through.

But more concerning still, you'll see:
Cardiac risk—valvulopathy.
Also risk of **pulmonary strain**,
So **echocardiograms** must remain.
Monitor the **heart** before and while,
With regular echoes in your file.
Track **growth, weight**, and **mood** each day,
And look for signs that drift astray.

Black box warning? Yes, it's clear:
For **heart valve disease**, we must steer
With frequent checks and close review—
This one needs a **structured view**.

Teach caregivers to measure true,
As **oral solution** must be due
By weight-based dosing, twice per round,
And **daily logs** should hold it down.

Controlled substance—Schedule IV,
Because of how it works in store.
Abuse is rare, but still a thought,
So every refill should be caught.
Drug interactions? Take care here:
Avoid with **SSRIs** or anything near
That boosts **serotonin** up too high—
Serotonin syndrome could apply.

So **Fintepla**, though niche and rare,
Brings hope to those in deep despair.
For seizures fierce and uncontrolled,
It brings a calm that's strong and bold.

GABAPENTIN (NEURONTIN)
Anticonvulsant / Neuropathic Pain Agent / GABA Analog

When **nerves misfire** or **burn with pain**,
And seizures travel through the brain,
Gabapentin lends its calming hand—
To help the storm inside you stand.
It looks like **GABA**, but here's the twist:
It **doesn't bind GABA**, it quietly assists.
Instead, it blocks **calcium flow**,
At **α2δ subunits**, nice and low.
It's used for **seizures**—partial type,
And **nerve pain** that's electric, ripe.
Like **diabetic neuropathy**, or shingles' flame,
It soothes the nerves that scream your name.
Side effects? A mellow bunch:
Drowsiness, dizziness, maybe a hunch
Of **edema, weight gain**, or **blurred thought**,
And **fatigue** more than you thought.
Rarely, **mood** may shift or fall,
So **suicide risk?** Still on the call.
Especially in those with mood decline,
Keep a **watchful mental line**.
Monitor kidney function well,
Because **renal dosing** breaks the spell.
And note: this drug must **taper slow**,
Or **withdrawal seizures** may overflow.

Teach patients: **space doses evenly**,
And don't take **with antacids recently**.
They should expect a **slow start rise**,
To lessen side effects that surprise.
No black box warning, but take care,
If **mood gets dark**, or thoughts despair.
And while abuse is fairly rare,
Some misuse it for a "floaty" air.
Drug interactions? Mostly chill—
But watch with **CNS depressants'** will.
It adds to **sleepiness** in the stack,
So avoid **opioids**, or dial them back.
So **Gabapentin**, chill and slow,
Brings down the pain, the nerve's wild glow.
Used with care and steady chart,
It helps the healing gently start.

GABAPENTIN ENACARBIL (HORIZANT)

Prodrug of Gabapentin / RLS & Postherpetic Neuralgia Agent

When **restless legs** won't let you sleep,
And **shingles pain** runs long and deep,
Gabapentin Enacarbil stands,
With **slow-release**, extended hands.
It's a **prodrug** form of **Gabapentin**,
Absorbed with **predictable intent**.
Converted in the gut with ease,
For **steady dosing**, meant to please.
Used for **restless legs syndrome** at night,
And **postherpetic neuralgia**'s bite.
It calms the nerves, smooths the flare,
And helps the legs stop kicking air.
It acts like **Gabapentin** still,
But offers more **controlled refill**.
Same **α2δ** binding trick,
To make the nerve fire less quick.
Side effects? A drowsy crew:
Somnolence, **dizziness**, stumbling too.
Fatigue, **blurred vision**, **swelling feet**,
And sometimes **suicidal retreat**.
Monitor for mood that shifts,
And **renal function** if it dips.
It's **once daily** for RLS folk,
At **5 PM**, with food, no joke.
Teach patients: **don't split or crush**,
And **no alcohol**—that's a rush.
Also warn of next-day haze,
So caution during driving days.
Black box warning? Not on file,
But **CNS effects** can last a while.
And misuse risk, while not extreme,
Has grown in some misuse routine.

Drug interactions? Just a few,
It's mostly clean in what it'll do.
But still beware **depressant blends**,
With **opioids**, the danger extends.
So **Horizant**, slow and long,
Brings RLS a quieter song.
It helps the nerves and pain subside,
With smoother waves and longer glide.

LAMOTRIGINE (LAMICTAL)
Antiepileptic / Mood Stabilizer / Sodium Channel Blocker

When **seizures spark** or **moods swing wide**,
And highs and lows are hard to hide,
Lamotrigine helps calm the wave—
A **steady shield**, both bright and brave.
It **blocks sodium channels**, slow and sure,
To help the neurons fire pure.
And in **bipolar** minds that rise and fall,
It softens mood swings, smooths them all.
Used for **partial** and **tonic-clonic** fight,
And **Lennox-Gastaut** both day and night.
In **bipolar depression**, too,
It lifts the lows while guarding you.
Side effects to note with care:
Dizziness, **headache**, vision glare.
Nausea, **tremor**, **sleepy tone**,
And mood swings if the dose is blown.
But here's the key—**go slow to start**,
Or **Stevens-Johnson** may break the heart.
A **rash** that spreads could be severe,
So titrate gently, once a year.
Black box warning? Yes—it's bold:
SJS and **TEN** can take hold.
So teach patients: **rash is not okay**—
Call your doctor right away.
Monitor for skin and mood,
Especially in the introlude.
And don't combine too fast with meds
That raise Lamictal in their threads.
Valproate especially slows the flow—
And doubles levels, nice and slow.
So when combined, use half the start,
To keep the skin from falling apart.
Teach patients: **don't skip doses** light,
Or start again without insight.
And **taper slow** if it must end,
To keep withdrawal from around the bend.
Drug interactions? Yes, a few:
Enzyme inducers pull it through.
Like **carbamazepine**—it clears it quick,
While **valproate** can make it stick
So **Lamotrigine**, with grace and might,
Brings seizure calm and mood insight.

LACOSAMIDE (VIMPAT)
Sodium Channel Modulator / Antiepileptic

When **neurons fire without control**,
And seizures threaten to take their toll,
Lacosamide helps calm the tide—
A **steady modulator** on your side.
It **enhances slow inactivation**,
Of **sodium channels** in the station.
Unlike the fast block many choose,
It lets the brain reset and cruise.
Used for **partial-onset seizures** first,
In adults and kids whose neurons burst.
Also now for **tonic-clonic flair**,
To help the brain find balanced air.
Side effects to watch and name:
Dizziness, nausea, double flame.
Fatigue, **diplopia**, and sometimes low
Coordination or **heart rate flow**.
Yes—**PR interval prolongation**,
Can lead to **arrhythmic complication**.
So **ECG** may be required,
If cardiac history is acquired.
Monitor for mood and mind,
As **suicidal thoughts** may unwind.
Track for **drowsiness**, **falls**, and swings,
And check how well seizure control clings.
Teach patients to **taper slow**,
Don't ever stop it on the go.
It comes as **tablet, liquid, IV**—
With flexibility for your strategy.
No black box warning, but stay aware,
If **conduction issues** linger there.
And always ask about the **heart**,
Before this med is set to start.
Drug interactions? Mild at most,
But **CNS depressants** share the host.
And combining with **antiarrhythmic drugs**,
Can increase risks with subtle shrugs.
So **Vimpat**, sleek and modern made,
Helps seizure storms begin to fade.
A careful guide in neural strife,
To guard the spark—and steady life.

LEVETIRACETAM (KEPPRA)
Antiepileptic / SV2A Modulator

When **seizures rise** without a sound,
And sparks in neurons spin around,
Levetiracetam takes control—
To help the brain regain its role.
It binds to **SV2A**,
A synaptic vesicle on display.
It **modulates neurotransmitter flow**,
To help that **excess firing slow**.
Used for **partial, tonic-clonic**, too,
And **myoclonic seizures** coming through.
It's safe for kids and grown-ups wide,
With dosing that can flex and slide.
Side effects? A modest set:
Fatigue, drowsiness, mood offset.
Irritability, agitation,
And rare **psychosis** or **hallucination**.
Though it's known to keep things calm,
Some feel an **emotional qualm**.
So **monitor mood**, and check in tight—
Especially if things don't feel right.
No black box warning, still beware
Of **suicidal thoughts** in the air.
Screen for history, check their view—
And always follow through.
Teach patients: take it **twice a day**,
With or without meals—either way.
Taper off if it must stop—
Or **rebound seizures** could suddenly pop.

Drug interactions? Pretty chill—
No CYP enzymes in its skill.
It plays well with most drug lines,
Which is rare in neuro signs.
But still, with other **CNS sedatives**,
It may enhance those sleepy relatives.
So warn about **alcohol** and **driving**,
While their system is still arriving.
So **Keppra**, simple, clean, and strong,
Keeps seizures from staying too long.
With stable dose and mindful track,
It helps the brain start fighting back.

LORAZEPAM IV (ATIVAN)
Benzodiazepine - Acute Seizure Management

In **seizure storms** that rage and shake, **IV Ativan** helps the body break. A **benzodiazepine**, fast and clear, To stop the waves of neural fear.

It binds to **GABA-A** with steady hand, Enhances **inhibition** as it's planned. Neurons slow, the firing fades, And consciousness begins to wade.

Used for **status epilepticus**, When two or more events erupt in us. Or when a seizure just won't end, This is the med that nurses send.

It works in **1 to 5 minutes fast**, And holds its calmness **longer than most last**. With less redistribution to the fat, It keeps the patient calm and flat.

Dosage depends on weight and age, Usually **4 mg IV** sets the stage. May repeat once if seizures go on, But **monitor breathing** till they're gone.

Respiratory depression is real and near, So keep **airway tools** and **oxygen** near. **Suction** ready, **reversal too**, In case the CNS shuts down on cue.

It may cause **hypotension**, so beware, And **sedation** may keep them unaware. **Dizziness**, **fatigue**, and **confusion** fit, So monitor closely as they sit.

It's used **short-term** and not for weeks, For **long-term use**, other methods it seeks. **Dependence risk** is fairly high, So taper slowly—don't just say goodbye.

In **elderly** or **hepatic strain**, Dose with caution, spare the brain. Monitor **LFTs**, keep tabs in place, And watch for falls in fragile space.

It's a **Schedule IV** in legal class, Stored in **secure kits** made to last. Must be charted right away, Controlled access — clear as day.

In **pregnancy**, the risks are real, But sometimes needed to help heal. If seizure harms both mom and child, Then **benefit outweighs the wild**.

So when a patient seizes strong, And you don't have very long, Reach for **Ativan IV** in haste— A med that brings the brain to grace.

OXCARBAZEPINE (TRILEPTAL)

Antiepileptic / Sodium Channel Blocker

When **neurons misfire**, fast and hot,
And **partial seizures** hit the spot,
Oxcarbazepine jumps in fast—
To calm the storm and make it last.
It **blocks sodium channels** with might,
To help the brain fire just right.
By stabilizing every spark,
It dims the waves that go too dark.
Used in **focal seizures**, young and old,
As **monotherapy** or with meds bold.
It's **well-tolerated**, clean and sleek,
With dosing **twice a day** each week.
Side effects? A few to name:
Dizziness, drowsiness, not too tame.
Nausea, double vision, fatigue,
And **ataxia** that can fatigue.
But here's the catch: in some, it lowers
Sodium levels—hyponatremia hovers.
So **monitor electrolytes**, just in case,
Especially in older face.
Rare but serious? **SJS** and rash—
So slow titration is key in the dash.
And watch for **mood** or **behavioral bend**,
As **suicide risk** may ascend.
Monitor sodium and mood swings wide,
And check for rashes that won't hide.
CBC and LFTs once in the mix,
Especially if they're on other picks.
Teach patients: take it **same time each day**,
Don't skip doses or toss it away.
Don't stop suddenly, **taper slow**,
Or seizures might begin to grow.
No black box warning, but beware
Of **skin reactions** and mental care.
And don't confuse with **Carbamazepine**—
It's different, though they share a theme.
Drug interactions? Yes, a few:
It's a **CYP inducer**, too.
May lower levels of **birth control**,
So back-up plans should play a role.
So **Trileptal**, calm and neat and true,
Helps seizures pause and pathways renew.

PERAMPANEL (FYCOMPA)
AMPA Receptor Antagonist / Antiepileptic

When **seizures surge** with sudden fire,
And neurons spark like tangled wire,
Perampanel steps in cool—
To **block excitatory fuel**.
It targets **AMPA receptors**, clear,
To calm the **glutamate** we fear.
By blocking these post-synaptic gates,
It slows the spread that overstimulates.
Used in **focal seizures**, solo or mix,
And **tonic-clonic** in the treatment fix.
It's once a day—**bedtime best**,
To sleep through side effects and rest.
Side effects? You'll need to track:
Dizziness, fatigue, gait thrown back.
Weight gain, irritability,
And sometimes **hostility.**
More rare—but watch for **mood unkind**,
Aggression, rage, and **darkened mind.**
Suicidal thoughts may rise,
So monitor for changing eyes.
Black box warning? Yes, it's there—
For **serious psych events**, beware.
Especially in teens or younger folk,
Where **rage or violence** may provoke.
Monitor behavior close,
Especially at higher dose.
And go slow—start low, titrate wise,
To help avoid those sharp surprise.
Teach patients: take it late,
With or without food on their plate.
Don't skip doses or stop abrupt—
That could cause seizures to erupt.
Drug interactions? Yes, for real—
With **enzyme inducers**, it may deal.
Like **carbamazepine** or **phenytoin**,
They drop levels, so keep checkin'.
So **Fycompa**, bold and fairly new,
Brings seizures down and thoughts back through.
But with great power must come care—
And close support from those who share.

PHENOBARBITAL (LUMINAL)

Barbiturate / Anticonvulsant / Sedative-Hypnotic

When **seizures rage** and won't let go,
And **CNS storms** run deep and low,
Phenobarbital calms the tide—
A **barbiturate** with power wide.
It binds to **GABA-A receptors' core**,
To **boost chloride** and calm the roar.
It **depresses neurons**, slows the brain,
To halt the seizure's pulsing chain.
Used for **tonic-clonic**, **focal**, and more,
Even for **status epilepticus** at the door.
It's old but strong, a classic name,
Still part of seizure's oldest game.
Side effects? A sleepy haze:
Sedation, ataxia, slowed-down phase.
Depression, confusion, and in youth,
It may delay their growth or truth.
Dependence risk is high and real—
So **withdrawal seizures** can reveal.
Respiratory depression comes,
Especially when **stacked with other drums**.
Black box warning? Yes, take note:
For **abuse** and **withdrawal's heavy coat**.
Stopping fast is not advised—
Taper slowly, keep supervised.
Monitor: blood levels, steady view,
Especially with polypharm crew.
Also track for **mood and drive**,
To help the patient truly thrive.

Teach patients: don't mix with drink,
And **caution driving**, pause and think.
It's long-acting, builds up slow,
But wears off late, so time it so.
Drug interactions? A major list—
It **induces CYPs**, can't be missed.
It lowers levels of many meds—
So check what's co-prescribed in threads.
So **Luminal**, with weight and grace,
Still holds a timeworn, steady place.
A sedative sword to stop the flame—
But best used wisely in the game.

PHENYTOIN (DILANTIN)
Anticonvulsant / Sodium Channel Blocker

When **neurons fire** in rapid storm,
And seizures break the brain's true form,
Phenytoin stands firm and tight—
To **stabilize** and set things right.
It blocks those **sodium channels fast**,
Keeping **action potentials** from being cast.
It stops the signal from spreading wide,
So seizures slow and waves subside.

Used in **tonic-clonic**, **focal**, too,
And sometimes post-**neurosurgery** view.
It's not the newest on the line—
But still a strong and steady spine.
Side effects? A loaded chest:
Nystagmus, **ataxia**, **tremors** at rest.
Gingival hyperplasia shows—
The **puffy gums** that overgrow.

Hirsutism, **rash**, and **skin may peel**,
With **Stevens-Johnson's** rare ordeal.
And **liver strain** or **blood count drops**,
So frequent labs help catch the stops.
Monitor: therapeutic range is key—
10 to 20 mcg/mL is where it should be.
Too low? Seizures. Too high? You'll find
Toxicity of the cerebellar kind.

Teach patients: don't skip a dose,
And **no sudden stop**—that's dangerous most.
Take with food, but not with milk,
And brush with care—gums aren't silk.
It's known for **nonlinear kinetics** bold,
A small dose rise? The levels unfold.
So dose with caution, slowly go,
Because plasma jumps can overflow.

Black box warning? Yes, it's true:
IV too fast can harm you.
Hypotension and **arrhythmias** live
When rates exceed what hearts can give.
Drug interactions? A tangled mess—
It's a **CYP inducer**, more or less.
It lowers many drug levels down,
From **warfarin** to **the pill**—watch that crown.

So **Dilantin**, with careful aim,
Still plays a role in seizure's game.
A powerful tool from days gone by,
But one to watch with a cautious eye.

PREGABALIN (LYRICA)
Anticonvulsant / Neuropathic Pain & Anxiety Agent / GABA Analog

When **nerves ignite** with burning fire,
And **fibro flares** refuse to tire,
Pregabalin steps in the scene,
To soothe the pain that's felt unseen.
It's not quite **GABA**, though it's close—
It binds to channels, calcium's post.
α2δ subunit is the name,
It tones down **neurotransmitter flame**.

Used for **neuropathy** and **seizures** mild,
And **fibromyalgia** pain compiled.
Also helps with **anxiety**,
Especially **off-label** in some decree.
Side effects? A sleepy flow:
Dizziness, fatigue, and **edema** grow.
Weight gain, blurred vision, dry mouth too,
And sometimes moods feel **low or blue**.

Monitor for swelling feet,
And signs of misuse on repeat.
Renal dosing needs adjustment fair—
It's excreted mostly out of there.
Teach patients: don't stop too fast,
Or **withdrawal symptoms** may come to pass.
It's **Schedule V**, a controlled line—
With **abuse potential**, though less than nine.

No black box warning, but don't ignore
Suicidal thoughts that knock the door.
Check for changes in the mind,
Especially in the anxious kind.
Drug interactions? Not a lot,
But with **CNS depressants**, watch the spot.
It may increase **sedation**, fall,
So don't mix freely, after all.

So **Lyrica**, with gentled thread,
Helps calm the pain that patients dread.
A steady nerve, a softer sound,
Where once the ache had held its ground.

PRIMIDONE (MYSOLINE)

Anticonvulsant / Barbiturate-Like / Essential Tremor & Seizure Agent

When **seizures spark** or **tremors shake**,
And hands won't calm with every break,
Primidone steps in the zone—
A med with roots in **barbitone**.
It's **converted in the liver's line**
To **phenobarbital** and **PEMA** in time.
So it calms the brain with **GABA's ease**,
To help the nerves find quiet and peace.
Used in **tonic-clonic seizures' ride**,
And **partial seizures** hard to hide.
It's also great for **tremor relief**,
Especially when **essential** shakes cause grief.
Side effects? A barbiturate blend:
Sedation, dizziness might not end.
Ataxia, nausea, and mental fog,
With **mood swings** sometimes in the log.
It may cause **blood dyscrasias**, rare,
Like **leukopenia**, so take care.
Rash, liver strain, or even more—
Monitor labs to track the score.
Teach patients to start it slow,
As sedation often steals the show.
Don't drive or drink while drowsy stays,
And warn of **withdrawal** if it strays.
Black box warning? Not per se,
But **dependency risk** may come to play.
It shares that **barbiturate gene**,
So **abuse potential** sits unseen.
Monitor: CBC, LFT,
And levels if toxicity you see.
Also track for **mood decline**,
Or suicidal warning sign.
Drug interactions? Yes, a crowd—
It's a **CYP inducer**, loud and proud.
It can reduce the drugs you pair—
So check your list with extra care.
So **Mysoline**, an older name,
Still holds a **valuable clinical claim**.
For seizures or for tremors bold,
It brings control, though a bit old.

PROPRANOLOL (INDERAL)

Non-Selective Beta Blocker / Antimigraine & Anxiolytic / Cardiovascular Agent

When **heartbeats race** and **tremors shake**,
And **migraine warnings** start to wake,
Propranolol steps in with care—
To **slow things down** and keep it fair.
It blocks both **beta-1 and 2**—
So **heart** and **lungs** are in its view.
By damping **sympathetic tone**,
It calms the nerves and guards the zone.

Used for **hypertension** and the heart,
Arrhythmias, and **angina's part**.
But in **neuro care**, it takes the stage
For **essential tremor** and **migraine rage**.
Also helps with **social fear**,
Performance shakes that disappear.
A steady pulse, a quiet mind,
In anxious types, it can be kind.

Side effects? A beta blend:
Bradycardia, where beats may end.
Fatigue, cold hands, dizzy states,
And **nightmares** through REM's fragile gates.
Bronchospasm is a risk—
Especially in **asthmatics**—so be brisk.
Avoid in those with **COPD**,
As blocking beta-2 shuts lungs, you see.

Monitor: BP, HR, and breath,
For signs of **slow or smothered depth**.
Check for **depression, blood sugar dips**,
It can **mask hypoglycemia's scripts**.
Teach patients not to stop too fast—
Or **rebound hypertension** may blast.
Take it with food to slow its pace,
And **space out doses** with steady grace.

No black box warning, but respect
Its power on the **cardiac circuit** deck.
And stack with care when CNS
Depressants may cause extra stress.
Drug interactions? Yes, indeed:
Calcium channel blockers may exceed.
And it may blunt the asthma meds,
Or hide the lows when sugar shreds.

So **Inderal**, though cardiac born,
Plays **neuro roles** from night to morn.
A beta-blocker, smooth and wide—
With calming strength and quiet pride

RUFINAMIDE (BANZEL)
Sodium Channel Modulator / Antiepileptic

When **seizures strike in Lennox style**,
And drop attacks come fast and wild,
Rufinamide steps in strong—
To help the brain **correct what's wrong**.
It's not fully clear how it works its art,
But it **modulates sodium channels** smart.
It helps control that misfired wave,
So patients may feel more behaved.
Used for **Lennox-Gastaut syndrome** first,
A seizure type that's often worst.
In kids and adults, it earns its place
As part of the **epilepsy brace**.
Side effects? A careful range:
Drowsiness, fatigue, and mood may change.
Nausea, vomiting, shortened QT,
And sometimes **rash** or **hostility**.
Multiorgan sensitivity—rare,
But still something to **monitor there**.
And **suicidal thoughts** can arise,
So track the patient's mental skies.
Monitor for seizures' rate,
And any signs that escalate.
LFTs, EKGs, weight gain or fall—
Especially if the patient's small.
Teach patients: take with food,
To help absorption and the mood.
Don't crush the tabs—**swallow whole**,
And taper down if that's the goal.
No black box warning, still use care,
When **behavior shifts** are in the air.
Watch for **hyperactivity**,
Especially in **children's activity**.
Drug interactions? There are some:
With **valproate**, the levels run.
CYP inducers (like phenytoin)
May drop its level in the joint.
So **Banzel**, for a seizure fight,
Helps bring **Lennox-Gastaut** some light.
Not first-line, but a steady tool,
In epilepsy's complex school.

TOPIRAMATE (TOPAMAX)
Anticonvulsant / Migraine Prophylaxis & Mood Stabilizer

When **seizures fire** or **migraines sting**,
And thoughts feel like a jumbled ring,
Topiramate comes in to play—
To keep those surges **held at bay**.
It's a **multi-action med**, quite rare:
Blocks **sodium channels**, trims the flare.
Enhances **GABA**, calms the brain,
While cutting **glutamate's** sharp pain.
Used for **epilepsy**, both wide and small,
Partial, tonic-clonic, it covers all.
Also used to **prevent migraines**,
And **bipolar lows** in mental lanes.
Off-label, it's seen in weight-loss crew,
And sometimes for **binge eating** too.
It's flexible—but not without
A side effect list worth thinking about.
Side effects? The famous fog:
Cognitive slowing, mental bog.
Tingling, drowsy, weight loss, yes,
And **word-finding trouble**—nonetheless.
Also: **kidney stones**—drink up, friend,
Hydration helps that trend to end.
Metabolic acidosis too,
So check those **bicarb labs** in view.
Monitor mood, and watch the frame,
As **suicidal thoughts** can claim.
And vision? Watch for something wrong—
Acute glaucoma doesn't take long.
Teach patients: titrate slow,
To keep side effects nice and low.
Twice a day, or XR style,
And taper if it's gone a while.
No black box warning, but proceed
With caution if there's **mental need**.
And caution with the pill you pick—
It **reduces birth control** pretty quick.
Drug interactions? Yes, a few:
It's **CYP-inducing** in its view.
And **valproate** may raise the risk
For **hypothermia** on the list.
So **Topamax**, both sharp and chill,
Brings calm where sparks would break the will.

VALPROIC ACID (DEPAKOTE)
Anticonvulsant / Mood Stabilizer / Migraine Prophylaxis

When **seizures fire**, or **moods swing wide**,
And thoughts are hard to **calm or guide**,
Valproic Acid takes the stage—
To stabilize the neural cage.
It **boosts GABA**, the brain's best friend,
And keeps those signals from reaching end.
It **blocks sodium** and calcium's flow,
So **neurons chill**, not overflow.
Used for **seizures**—all kinds in line:
Tonic-clonic, absence, and others in time.
Also helps in **bipolar lows**,
And **migraine prevention**, as science shows.
Side effects? A hefty crew:
Nausea, weight gain, tremor, too.
Hair loss, sleepiness, GI strife,
And **PCOS risk** in reproductive life.
Serious risks are not so rare—
Hepatotoxicity, so beware.
And **pancreatitis**, sudden and deep,
With **abdominal pain** that doesn't sleep.
And in **pregnancy**, it's a line to fear—
Neural tube defects are crystal clear.
So it's **black box warned** (yes, it's true)
For **fetal harm**, and **liver damage**, too.
Monitor: LFTs, CBC,
And **serum levels** routinely.
Also track **ammonia high**,
As **hyperammonemia** may apply.
Teach patients: take with food,
To ease the stomach's edgy mood.
Don't crush **ER tabs**, and know the signs
Of **toxicity** crossing lines.
Drug interactions? Yes, a stack—
It plays with many drugs, in fact.
It **inhibits liver enzymes** strong,
So **lamotrigine** won't last long.
So **Depakote**, bold and widely known,
Helps minds and neurons find their tone.
But always used with eyes on guard—
For **risks and benefits** must be weighed hard.

VIGABATRIN (SABRIL)
GABA Transaminase Inhibitor / Antiepileptic

When **seizures start** and won't let go,
And **infantile spasms** steal the show,
Vigabatrin steps in bold—
To help the storm lose hold.
It **inhibits GABA transaminase**,
So **GABA levels** rise and stay.
More calming signals flood the brain,
To **quiet seizures**, ease the strain.
Used for **infantile spasms**, clear,
And **refractory focal seizures** near.
Especially for **Tuberous Sclerosis** kind,
Where few other meds align.
Side effects? A major one:
Permanent vision loss can be done.
Black box warning, loud and plain—
Visual field defects that remain.
Eye exams are a must before,
And **every 3-6 months** once more.
But even then, there is no sure
Prevention from this optic blur.
Other effects? There may be:
Sedation, irritability,
Weight gain, fatigue, and mood swings fast—
And **MRI changes** that may not last.
Monitor: vision first and most,
And **neuro status**—don't just coast.
Also check for **psych effects**,
Like **psychosis, agitation,** and **suicide checks**.
Teach patients: risk is real,
But so is **seizure-free appeal**.

Start low, go slow, then rise in kind—
And taper off or you'll rewind.
Drug interactions? Not too wide,
But **decreases phenytoin** on the side.
And combos with **CNS meds** may
Make drowsiness or mood delay.
So **Sabril**, potent, serious, rare,
Is used when options aren't all there.
A rescue med with vision cost,
That gives back peace, but not without loss.

ZONISAMIDE (ZONEGRAN)

Anticonvulsant / Sulfonamide Derivative / Broad-Spectrum Seizure Agent

When **seizures spike** in random fire,
And brains miswire or misfire,
Zonisamide steps in the frame—
To help the sparks forget their game.
It **blocks sodium channels** with control,
And slows **T-type calcium** in its role.
Plus it **modulates GABA**, too—
A triple threat to seizures through.
Used for **partial seizures** in the mix,
Adjunct therapy in adult picks.
Sometimes off-label, though not core,
For **bipolar** and **migraine** lore.
Side effects? A subtle tide:
Drowsiness, dizziness, fog inside.
Weight loss, loss of appetite,
And sometimes **kidney stones** at night.
It may impair the body's cool—
So warn of **heatstroke** as a rule.
Especially in **kids**, who play in heat,
This side effect is no small feat.
Rare but real? Metabolic sway—
Like **acidosis** along the way.
So check **bicarb** levels, **watch their tone**,
Especially if they're feeling thrown.
Teach patients: don't stop fast—
Taper slowly, make it last.
Hydrate well to keep stones gone,
And report confusion if it dawns.
No black box warning, but beware
Of mood changes floating in the air.
Suicidal thoughts, though rare,
Still deserve provider care.

Drug interactions? Quite a few—
It's metabolized by **CYP3A4** too.
It may play with **enzyme inducers**,
And lower levels in its users.
Also: it's a **sulfa drug**,
So if they're allergic—pull the plug.
Skin rashes, fevers, organ strain—
Allergic reactions bring the pain.
So **Zonegran**, quiet, sleek, and wide,
Brings balance back to neuron tide.

ns & Movement
Part II Parkinson's & Movement Disorders

AMANTADINE (SYMMETREL, GOCOVRI)
Dopamine Promoter / Antiviral Agent

Once made for **flu**, now finds its lane,
In **Parkinson's** and **movement pain**.
Amantadine, a helper neat,
For tremors, **rigid limbs**, and shuffled feet.
It boosts up **dopamine's release**,
And blocks its **reuptake**, piece by piece.
Also **NMDA antagonism** plays,
Reducing **dyskinesia** in subtle ways.

Indications? Let's review:
Parkinson's, early or as add-on too.
Helps with **drug-induced EPS**,
And still used for the flu—though less.
Side effects you'll need to spot:
Livedo reticularis—purple blot.
Dry mouth, blurred vision, hallucination,
Confusion, swelling, constipation.

Orthostatic hypotension might show,
So rise up **slowly**, take it slow.
Can also cause **impulse drives**,
Like risky spending or wild vibes.
Monitor the mental state,
And **renal function**—don't be late.
Reduce the dose if **kidneys lag**,
And keep an eye for that **purple rash tag**.

Teach patients how to **rise with care**,
And watch for moods that aren't quite fair.
Report **swelling**, mood changes too,
Or if the skin has a **mottled hue**.
No **black box warning**, but be wise,
It's not for kids with **seizure ties**.
Avoid with other **dopaminergic blends**,
And **anticholinergics**, lest chaos ascends.

So **Amantadine**, an old-school gem,
Brings movement back to stiffened limbs.
Use it right, and you will see,
A smoother path for neurology.

APOMORPHINE (APOKYN)

Dopamine Agonist

When **Parkinson's** brings a sudden freeze,
And movement halts like locked-up knees,
Apomorphine jumps to play,
To get them moving right away.
A **dopamine agonist**, fast and true,
It **stimulates D2 receptors** through and through.
It mimics dopamine's lost song,
To right the wrongs that last too long.

Used for **rescue in off episodes**,
When meds wear off and stiffness loads.
It works **subQ**, with rapid fire—
A lifeline when the limbs retire.
But oh, the **side effects** may bite:
Nausea, **vomiting**, quite the plight.
Yawning, **drowsy**, **hallucination**,
Low BP and **injection irritation**.

To help prevent the **GI war**,
They often give **trimethobenzamide** before.
(Not for **ondansetron**—it's banned here,
That mix can bring a heart arrhythmia near.)
Monitor for syncope and fall,
And **QT changes**—track them all.
Rotate injection spots with care,
And screen for **cardiac issues** there.

Teach patients how to **self-inject**,
With signs of **hypotension** to detect.
It acts **within 10 minutes flat**,
So have them sit—and grab a mat!
No **black box**, but still proceed
With caution, dosing, and patient need.
Avoid with other **dopaminergic drugs**,
And beware of **serotonin syndrome bugs**.

So **Apomorphine**, though short and quick,
Can turn the key when symptoms stick.
With patient guidance, skill, and prep,
It brings their step back into step.

APOMORPHINE SUBLINGUAL (KYNMOBI)
Dopamine Agonist – Parkinson's OFF Episodes

When tremors strike and **meds wear thin**, And Parkinson's fights from deep within, **Kynmobi** comes beneath the tongue, A **quick relief** for brains unsprung.

A **dopamine agonist** by class, It mimics what the brain can't pass. It binds to **D2 receptors** fast, And helps the **"off" time** not to last.

Used when **carbidopa's** effects fade, This **rescue med** is quickly laid. It **bypasses the gut**, no food delay— A **sublingual strip** that saves the day.

It kicks in fast — in **10 to 20**, To turn the motor back to plenty. So speech returns, and gait resumes, Instead of silence, stares, and gloom.

Yet **nausea** strikes with brutal flair, So give a **trimethobenzamide** pair. Start antiemetics **three days before**, Or vomiting might hit the floor.

Other effects to watch with care: **Yawning, drowsy, orthostatic flare**. **Hallucinations** may appear, So don't give it without clear fear.

It's **not for daily symptom control**, But for **rescue use**, it plays its role. Only **two doses** in a day, And **six hours apart**, come what may.

Avoid in patients with **lung disease**, Or low BP that drops with ease. It can **depress the breath or chest**, So screen your patients to assess.

Under the tongue, it quickly goes, But wait to eat till swelling slows. **Irritation**, **mouth pain**, and more, May make patients their docs implore.

Teach how to place and **time the dose**, And wait for full **effect to close**. Avoid with **5HT3 antagonists**, too— Like **Zofran**, which could harm you.

Not a first-line dopamine start, But useful when the symptoms dart. So keep **Kynmobi** close at hand, To **bridge the gap** when things get out of hand.

BENZTROPINE (COGENTIN)

Anticholinergic / Antiparkinsonian Agent

When **tremors shake** and **rigid limbs** hold tight,
Benztropine steps in to fight.
An **anticholinergic**, smooth and sly,
It helps those **Parkinson's** symptoms die.
It blocks **acetylcholine's grip**,
To let that **dopamine** re-equip.
Restores the balance in the brain,
To ease the shake, the muscle strain.
Used for **Parkinson's**, sure—but more!
For **EPS** from antipsychotic war.
It calms the **dystonia**, stops the twitch,
And helps the **neuroleptic glitch**.
Side effects? The classic crew:
Dry mouth, **blurry vision**, bowel backup too.
Urinary retention, **confusion**, heat—
And **sedation** that might knock you off your feet.
In **older adults**, beware the haze—
It might ignite **delirium's maze**.
Watch for **hallucinations**, mental slide,
And always keep the **fall risk** in mind.
Monitor intake and output counts,
And signs of **retention** that mount.
Watch for **fever**—can't sweat it out,
Heatstroke risk is real—no doubt.
Teach patients: avoid the sun,
Stay **hydrated** till the day is done.
Don't stop quick—taper low,
Or **Parkinson's symptoms** may overflow.

No **black box warning**, but still take care,
Especially in those **with glaucoma glare**.
Avoid in **BPH** or memory loss,
This med comes with a subtle cost.
Interactions? Yes, a few—
With **antihistamines**, **TCA** too.
Other **anticholinergics** can clash,
And ramp up side effects in a flash.
So **Benztropine**, though small in name,
Can settle nerves and calm the flame.
Use it wisely, dose with grace,
To bring control to a trembling space.

CARBIDOPA/LEVODOPA (SINEMET)

Dopamine Precursor + Decarboxylase Inhibitor

When **Parkinson's** slows the body's beat,
And shuffling steps can't find their feet,
Sinemet steps in with grace,
To **bring back dopamine's embrace**.
Levodopa—a **precursor true**,
Turns into **dopamine** like it used to do.
But in the gut, it breaks too fast—
So **Carbidopa** helps it last.
Carbidopa **blocks the breakdown** early,
So more gets past the **GI hurly-burly**.
It also lessens side effect scenes—
Like **nausea**, **vomit**, and belly means.
This combo treats the **motor signs**:
Bradykinesia, rigid spines,
Tremors, freezing, gait that drags—
It gives the brain its missing flags.
Side effects may still appear:
Dyskinesia, or twitching near.
Nausea, orthostatic lows,
Hallucinations as the dose grows.
Long-term use can bring some tricks:
Like **on-off swings** and **wearing-off kicks**.
So monitor for these changes clear,
And tweak the schedule year by year.

Check for **mental shifts or mood**,
And dose with **food**—but not high-protein food!
(Too much **protein** fights absorption,
Leading to motor disruption.)
Teach patients: timing is key,
And report any odd **compulsivity**.
Like **gambling, shopping**, urges strange—
Impulse control may rearrange.
No **black box warning**, but still, be wise,
This med affects both brain and thighs.
It interacts with **MAOIs**,
And **antipsychotics** may paralyze.
So **Carbidopa/Levodopa**, gold standard still,
Brings movement back with skill and will.
Treats the tremor, smooths the way—
With careful use, it saves the day.

ENTACAPONE (COMTAN)
COMT Inhibitor / Parkinson's Disease Adjunct

When **Levodopa** starts to fade too fast,
And **"off" time** seems to always last,
Entacapone joins the team,
To help extend dopamine's dream.
A **COMT inhibitor**, it blocks the way
Levodopa **breaks down too soon each day**.
By stopping COMT's degradin' spree,
It helps the brain get dopamine free.
It's **not used alone**—but side-by-side,
With **Carbidopa/Levodopa** as your guide.
For **Parkinson's**, it smooths the ride,
And keeps that movement from the slide.
Side effects are worth the glance:
Diarrhea, dyskinesia, may enhance.
Nausea, confusion, hallucination,
Or even **urine discoloration**!
It might turn **orange, red, or brown**—
But it's harmless, so don't frown.
Still, **liver enzymes** should be screened,
Though less than older COMT scene.
Monitor for mental changes new,
And how much **"on time"** breaks on through.
Track for **fall risk**, sudden jerks,
As **Levodopa's effects** may work in bursts.

Teach patients this is **added on**,
Not a solo drug to lean upon.
Take **with each dose** of their main pill,
To stretch the dopamine refill.
No black box warning, but take care,
If **diarrhea** is severe—beware.
Could point to **colitis** in disguise,
So notify the team that's wise.
Drug interactions? Mostly mild,
But **other COMT drugs** are reconciled.
And with **dopaminergic meds**, the tone
May lead to **too much dopamine zone**.
So **Entacapone**, with subtle might,
Helps keep **Parkinson's tremors light**.
A sidekick med with solid grace,
To help the brain keep up the pace.

PRAMIPEXOLE (MIRAPEX)

Dopamine Agonist / Parkinson's Disease & Restless Legs Syndrome Agent

When **dopamine dips** and movements stall,
And **Parkinson's tremors** start to sprawl,
Pramipexole joins the quest—
To help the brain feel more at rest.
It's a **dopamine agonist**, light and clean,
That mimics D_2 in the scene.
It also hits D_3 with grace,
To **lift the mood** and **steady pace**.
Used for **Parkinson's**, early and late,
To help with **rigid gait and gait**.
Also treats **restless legs at night**,
To help the limbs stop kicking fight.
Side effects? A tricky crew:
Nausea, dizziness, sleepiness too.
Hallucinations, impulse drive,
Like **gambling, shopping**, taken in stride.
Orthostatic hypotension may start,
So monitor with a gentle heart.
And note the risk of **sudden sleep**,
Where waking minds may dive too deep.
Monitor: behavior, sleep, and sway—
Especially in the **elderly gray**.
Track for **mood** and **hallucination**,
And check in with each titration.
Teach patients: start **low and slow**,
Then rise as symptoms come and go.
If they stop, **don't restart full**,
Titrate again so things stay cool.

No black box warning, but take care,
With **impulse control**, be aware.
And caution when combining near
Other meds that hit dopamine's gear.
Drug interactions? A modest set—
With **sedatives**, the sleep risk's met.
And with **antipsychotics**, effects may dull,
Since dopamine's the game they pull.
So **Mirapex**, with mimic grace,
Brings **balance back to time and space**.
A steady guide through tremor's trail,
To help the strength of mind prevail.

RASAGILINE (AZILECT)
MAO-B Inhibitor / Parkinson's Disease Agent

When **dopamine fades** and tremors grow,
And **Parkinson's pace** begins to slow,
Rasagiline steps in with grace—
To help extend that **dopamine space**.
It's a **monoamine oxidase-B blocker**,
Keeps dopamine from the breakdown locker.
By stopping **MAO-B's** hungry bite,
It helps the motor sparks ignite.
Used alone in **early stage**,
Or added in the **later page**.
It smooths the ride with **levodopa**,
And cuts down on the **"off-time" slope-a**.
Side effects? Usually light:
Headache, joint pain, insomnia's night.
Some may feel **nausea, dizzy slips**,
Or **orthostatic BP dips**.
More rarely: **serotonin storm**—
If mixed with meds that **boost that form**.
So **SSRIs, tramadol, St. John's Wort**
Could send things veering off report.
Monitor for mood and mind,
And signs of **hypertension kind**.
Though **MAO-B** is selective here,
At high doses, that line's not clear.
Teach patients: watch what they eat—
Aged cheese, meats, and wine so sweet.

Though **less restrictive** than MAO-A,
Tyramine can still cause dismay.
No black box warning, but don't ignore
The risk of stacking serotonin more.
And in combo with **levodopa's lift**,
May raise **dyskinesia**—a motor shift.
Drug interactions? Yes, proceed
With caution if **psych meds** are in the feed.
And always ask before they start
A new RX that plays with the heart.
So **Azilect**, quiet, smooth, and wise,
Helps **dopamine levels** stabilize.
A once-daily boost to movement's flow,
Helping **Parkinson's pace** go slow.

ROPINIROLE (REQUIP)

Dopamine Agonist / Parkinson's Disease & Restless Legs Syndrome Agent

When **legs won't rest** or **tremors grow**,
And **dopamine levels** dip too low,
Ropinirole joins the plan—
To mimic what the brain began.
A **dopamine agonist**, smooth and bright,
It binds to **D$_2$ receptors** tight.
It helps with **movement**, calm and clear,
In **Parkinson's** and **RLS** gear.
Used for **early PD alone**,
Or **with levodopa** later shown.
For **restless legs**, it's often tried
To keep the twitching things inside.
Side effects? Some might feel:
Drowsiness, nausea, dizzy wheel.
Orthostatic hypotension, too,
And **sudden sleep attacks**—rare but true.
Impulse control can go astray—
Like **gambling, spending, sex**, or play.
So screen for risks and check in deep,
Especially if they don't get sleep.
Monitor BP, mental state,
And how they walk, eat, sleep, or wait.
Mood shifts, **hallucinations** may show,
Especially as the doses grow.
Teach patients: titrate slow,
To keep side effects nice and low.
Take with food if **nausea plays**,
And **bedtime dosing** helps in RLS phase.
No black box warning, but be smart—
Track how it plays on mind and heart.
Avoid quick stops—**taper down**,
Or withdrawal symptoms may come around.
Drug interactions? Not a crowd,
But **CYP1A2** should be allowed.
Ciprofloxacin can raise its ride,
So dose adjustments may coincide.
So **Requip**, calm and dopamine-bright,
Brings motion back and rest at night.
A quiet helper, smooth and wide,
To walk again with strength and pride.

ROPINIROLE ER (REQUIP XL)

Dopamine Agonist - Restless Legs & Parkinson's

When legs won't stop and sleep won't stay, And **restless nights** steal peace away, **Ropinirole ER** steps in, To calm the nerves beneath the skin.

A **dopamine agonist** in class, It helps those surges slowly pass. It binds **D2 receptors** tight, To **ease the urge** and stop the fight.

Approved for **RLS**, it soothes the twitch, The creepy-crawly, jumpy glitch. And in **Parkinson's**, it may serve, When **"off" time** throws the motor curve.

The **ER form** lasts through the night, With **steady dosing** — no quick spike. One **daily dose**, no need to split, A smoother curve with lesser hit.

Side effects that may appear: **Drowsiness, dizzy, nausea,** fear. **Hallucinations, compulsive need**, To **gamble, shop,** or **overfeed**. **Orthostatic drops** may show, So rise up slowly, take it slow. And watch for **sleep attacks**, abrupt— They're rare but sudden, so heads up.

Dose it **low**, then titrate slow, Let tolerance and time both grow. Don't stop fast—**taper it with care**, Or symptoms may come back unfair.

It's metabolized by **CYP1A2**, So don't mix **ciprofloxacin** in that stew. Smoking can reduce effect, So assess each habit and suspect.

Not a cure, but **symptom ease**, It brings the jumping legs some peace. And helps the **dopamine** restore Its flow in brains that struggle more. So if the night feels sharp and long, And legs just won't behave or belong, Then **Ropinirole ER** may be A nightly route to tranquility.

ROTIGOTINE (NEUPRO)
Dopamine Agonist / Parkinson's Disease & Restless Legs Syndrome Agent

When **dopamine fades** and movement stalls
And **rigid limbs** ignore your calls,
Rotigotine comes through the skin,
To bring the **dopamine back in**.
A **dopamine agonist**, nice and slow,
It binds to **D$_1$, D$_2$, D$_3$** in flow.
Delivered via **transdermal patch**,
It gives a **steady 24-hour batch**.

Used for **Parkinson's**, early through late,
And **restless legs** that agitate.
It helps with **gait, rigidity**, and more—
While skipping pills you'd swallow before.
Side effects? A classic few:
Nausea, drowsiness, maybe **flu**.
Site reactions—itch or red,
And sometimes **dreams that fill the head**.

Hallucinations, low BP,
And sudden sleep attacks may be.
Plus **impulse issues** might arise—
Like **gambling, sex**, or spending highs.
Monitor: mental state and skin,
And how their motor symptoms spin.
Blood pressure, weight, and mood as well—
Especially if side effects swell.

Teach patients: patch goes **once a day**,
To clean, dry, hairless skin—okay?
Avoid heat, don't cut or bend,
And **rotate sites** to let skin mend.
If stopped, don't pull off and quit—
Taper slowly, bit by bit.
And caution if they live alone—
Sleep attacks strike without a moan.

No black box warning, but take care
In elders, **psychosis** may flare.
And **renal or hepatic strain**
May need adjustment in the chain.
Drug interactions? Mild and light,
But **dopaminergic stacking** might
Increase the risk for dyskinesia—
So dose with balance, not amnesia.

So **Neupro**, sleek and patch-applied,
Helps movement smooth and limbs abide.
For tremors, stiffness, legs at night—
It brings the brain a little light.

SAFINAMIDE (XADAGO)
MAO-B Inhibitor / Parkinson's Disease Adjunct Therapy

When **"off" times come** and tremors creep,
And **levodopa's boost** falls steep,
Safinamide steps in with flair—
To help bring movement **back with care.**
It's a **MAO-B inhibitor**, clean and bright,
That keeps **dopamine** in the light.
But it does more than just that lane—
It **blocks glutamate** to **calm the brain.**

Used for **Parkinson's disease on top,**
When **levodopa's power starts to drop.**
It extends the **"on" time**, smooths the gaps,
And helps reduce those motor traps.
Side effects? A manageable few:
Dyskinesia may rise in view.
Falls, nausea, and **insomnia,**
Sometimes **hypertension** might draw.

Rare, but note: **serotonin surge**
If other meds with it converge.
So with **SSRIs**, keep the dose mild,
And watch the patient's mood and style.
No black box warning, but take care
With **hepatic issues** anywhere.
It's **contraindicated** if **liver's late,**
So check LFTs before you gate.

Teach patients: take it once a day,
With or without meals, okay.
Usually started at **50 mg,**
Then **100 mg** if symptoms drag.
Drug interactions? Yes, for sure—
Avoid **MAOIs** or trouble's in store.
And steer away from **dextromethorphan,**
Or **tramadol**, which could go wrong.

So **Xadago**, steady, small, and wise,
Helps **Parkinson's patients** mobilize.
With dopamine preserved and flow refined,
It brings the strength to move the mind.

SELEGILINE (ELDEPRYL, ZELAPAR)

MAO-B Inhibitor / Parkinson's Disease & Depression Agent

When **dopamine fades** and motion slows,
And **Parkinson's disease** more clearly shows,
Selegiline lends its helping hand,
To keep that signal **strong and planned**.
It's a **selective MAO-B block**,
That slows **dopamine's metabolic clock**.
It helps preserve the brain's supply,
So patients move with less good-bye.
Used in **early PD**, alone,
Or **with levodopa** later shown.
It may reduce the need for more,
And smooth those **"off" times** patients store.
Zelapar melts on the tongue just right,
Eldepryl comes in tabs for bite.
It's also used—though less today—
For **depression** in a transdermal way.
Side effects? A light parade:
Insomnia, since **it can excite** the brain cascade.
Nausea, dizziness, sometimes mood,
And rare **serotonin syndrome** too, if stacked with certain food.
Teach patients: tyramine still may Cause **hypertensive storms** in play—
Though risk is low at **PD dose**,
High amounts can still be gross.
Black box warning? In the patch,
For **antidepressant risks** that match.
Suicidal thoughts in young adults Require care and close consults.
Monitor mood, BP, and sleep,
And tremors if they start to creep.
If used with **levodopa**, beware—
Dyskinesias may fill the air.
Drug interactions? Yes, a few:
SSRIs, meperidine, too.
Avoid with **MAO-A inhibitors**,
And **triptans**—they're potential critters.
So **Selegiline**, light and wise,
Extends **dopamine's hopeful rise**.
A small med with a pointed role,
To help the body and brain feel whole.

SELEGILINE PATCH (EMSAM)
MAOI - Transdermal Antidepressant

A patch that lifts the dark and gloom, **Emsam** works without a pill's perfume. A **transdermal MAOI**, It boosts the brain and lifts the sky. **Selegiline**, in oral form, Is used for **Parkinson's** to perform. But here, its purpose isn't that— It treats **depression**, flat and flat.

It blocks **monoamine oxidase B**, To keep **dopamine**, **serotonin** free. And at higher doses, **MAO-A** too, Letting **norepinephrine** pull through.

By bypassing the **gut and liver**, It reduces risks that often shiver. No first-pass route, so steady stream— The patch provides a smoother beam.

At **6 mg**, there's **no food concern**, But higher doses shift the turn. If **9 or 12**, you must avoid Tyramine foods that can't be toyed.

No **aged cheese**, no **fermented brew**, Or **hypertensive crisis** may ensue. The **"cheese effect"** is well-defined— So warn your patients, be aligned.

Side effects may still appear: **Insomnia**, **dizziness**, even fear. **Headache**, **dry mouth**, loss of weight, And rare but real, a risky state.

Watch out for **serotonin storm**, If mixed with meds outside the norm— Like **SSRIs**, **tramadol**, or more, Discontinue them days before.

Apply to **torso**, clean and dry, Rotate the site, and do not lie. No heat packs near or sauna tricks— That can increase how fast it sticks.

It's not for those with **seizure risk**, Or kids and teens — they must resist. And **bipolar patients** should be screened, Or mania may intervene.

It's reserved for **MDD**, When others fail to set you free. **Atypical**, but worth the shot, When stubborn sadness ties the knot.

So when the pills just won't engage, And mood is trapped within a cage, Consider **Emsam**, patch applied— A novel way to lift the tide.

TOLCAPONE (TASMAR)
COMT Inhibitor - Parkinson's Disease

When **dopamine** starts to decay, And **Parkinson's** steals strength away, Add **Tolcapone** to hold the line— A **COMT inhibitor** by design.
It blocks **catechol-O-methyltransferase**, Which breaks down **levodopa** fast. So more remains to cross the brain, And ease the tremor, slow the strain.
It's **never used alone** or first, But with **carbidopa/levodopa** bursts. Together, they prolong the dose, And keep the **"off-time"** less verbose.
Compared to **Entacapone**, It lasts much longer on its own. But that comes with a **heavier cost**— The **risk of liver being lost**.
Hepatotoxicity leads the chart, So test **LFTs** right from the start. Check at baseline, then again— Every two weeks, then widen the span.
If **ALT or AST** rise, Or **bilirubin** multiplies, **Discontinue without delay**, And call the doctor right away.
Watch for **dyskinesias** that may rise, As more levodopa fills the skies. Also note **diarrhea, nausea, sleep,** And **confusion** in the deep.
It's taken **three times every day, Before the meals**—that's the way. But due to risk, it's not preferred, Just held in case it's truly stirred.
It's contraindicated in those with **Liver disease** or a **history** myth. So screen with care before you start, This drug can truly harm the heart.

If switching from **Entacapone**, Don't overlap—give time alone. Always **educate** with truth and grace, So patients know it's not first place.
Used with caution, rarely bold, It's power wrapped in careful hold. But for some with **off-time wide**, **Tolcapone** helps the brain decide.

TRIHEXYPHENIDYL (ARTANE)

Anticholinergic / Parkinson's Disease & Drug-Induced Extrapyramidal Symptom Agent

When **rigid limbs** won't glide with ease,
And **tremors shake** in Parkinson's tease,
Trihexyphenidyl takes its place—
To calm the nerves and smooth the pace.
It blocks **acetylcholine's command**,
So **dopamine** can better stand.
By tipping back the balance lost,
It soothes the **shakes** at modest cost.
Used in **Parkinson's** early phase,
Or when **antipsych meds** misbehave.
It treats those **EPS effects**—
Like **dystonia, rigid necks**.
Side effects? The anticholinergic kind:
Dry mouth, blurred vision, foggy mind.
Constipation, urinary delay,
And **heat intolerance** in the day.
Confusion may appear in time,
Especially in the **elderly climb**.
And **memory lapses** might arise,
So screen for risks behind the eyes.
Monitor: cognition, mood, and gait,
Especially when **fall risks** elevate.
Teach patients: hydrate, stay cool,
And don't skip doses as a rule.
Taper slowly if you quit,
Or **withdrawal** may throw a fit.
And best to **take with food** or snack,
To avoid the GI grumble back.

No black box warning, still beware—
In older folks, use with care.
For **delirium, falls**, or mental slide,
It may do more than just subside.
Drug interactions? Yes indeed:
With **other anticholinergics**, it may exceed.
And **CNS depressants** may combine,
To cloud the brain or slow the spine.
So **Artane**, though a vintage tool,
Still plays a part in movement school.
With tremors tamed and stiffness eased,
It helps the motor storm be teased.

ISTRADEFYLLINE (NOURIANZ)

Adenosine A2A Receptor Antagonist / Parkinson's Disease Adjunct

When **Parkinson's meds** begin to fail
And **"off" times** make the progress stale,
Istradefylline adds its spark—
To help the movement find its mark.
It's not a **dopamine-type fix**,
But works within the basal mix.
It blocks **adenosine A2A**,
Which helps the motor circuits play.
Used to treat those **"off" episodes**,
When **Levodopa** alone explodes
Into a stop-and-start routine—
This med helps make the shifts more clean.
Side effects? Some may find:
Dyskinesia, more movement grind.
Also **hallucinations**, **insomnia**,
Or **dizziness** and **nausea**.
Impulse control may rise again,
So track for **gambling**, **spending**, or **sin**.
Mood shifts, **psychosis**, confusion's drift—
So monitor for any mental shift.
No black box warning, but beware
In those with **psych symptoms** in the air.
And while **renal safe**, use care with **liver**,
As severe disease makes dosing shiver.
Monitor how "on" time grows,
And if **dyskinesia** overflows.
Check how well it blends with base—
Most still need **Levodopa's grace**.

Teach patients it's not for start,
But **add-on** when the gaps break heart.
Take once a day—**with or without food**,
But check for **insomnia**, if it intrudes.
Drug interactions? CYP1A2's the key—
So watch for **Ciprofloxacin** tea.
Also smokers may clear it fast,
So higher doses may be cast.
So **Nourianz**, though not first-line,
Can help smooth out the motor spine.
With steady use and thoughtful track,
It helps bring **"on" time** safely back.

Part III
Multiple Sclerosis & Autoimmune Neuro Meds

ALEMTUZUMAB (LEMTRADA)

Monoclonal Antibody – Anti-CD52

A **monoclonal antibody**, sleek and bold,
It targets **CD52**, we're told.
Wipes out **T and B cells** fast,
To slow **MS relapses** that often last.
It's for **relapsing MS**, not first in line—
But used when others don't work fine.
It calms the fire, resets the fight,
Yet brings some risks—so dose it right.

Side effects may take a toll:
Infusion reactions top the scroll.
Rash, fever, and **thyroid flare**,
Even **autoimmune issues**—beware.
There's risk of **infections**, some quite grim,
UTIs, herpes, and **fungal within**.
Plus **malignancy** could take stage,
So screen with care at every age.

Monitor labs before each round:
CBC, creatinine, all must be sound.
And monthly labs for **4 years** post-last dose,
Because delayed issues come the most.
Teach patients to **avoid live vaccines**,
And signs of **infection**—know what that means.
Report **bleeding, bruising**, or feeling low,
And **thyroid shifts**—let your nurses know!

Black box warnings? Yes, a few:
Malignancy, autoimmunity, and **infusion stew**.
Only give in centers prepared,
Where **emergent care** is well declared.
Drug interactions? Don't combine
With other **immunosuppressants** in line.
Avoid **live vaccines** during and after,
To prevent complications or disaster.

So **Alemtuzumab**, strong and rare,
Needs skilled hands and lots of care.
It fights MS when others fall,
But watch your labs, and heed the call.

CLADRIBINE (MAVENCLAD)
Immunosuppressant / Purine Antimetabolite

For **MS** that keeps returning strong,
When other meds don't last too long,
Cladribine takes a deeper route—
It knocks those **lymphocytes** right out.
A **purine analog**, sly and small,
It **interferes with DNA** call.
It's toxic to **B and T cell troops**,
Reducing their autoimmune loops.
It treats **relapsing MS types** bold—
Not for **mild** or **benign**, we're told.
A short-course pill, just **2 years'** span,
But impacts stretch beyond that plan.
Side effects need careful eyes:
Infections, lymphopenia may rise.
Headache, nausea, fatigue may stay,
And **herpes zoster** might find a way.
Most concerning: **malignancy**—
So screen with **cancer history**.
Also risk of **PML**, though rare,
That brain infection needs some care.
Monitor CBCs before and after,
And **renal** labs to avoid disaster.
Check for **HIV**, **TB**, and **hep B**—
Infections can rise invisibly.
Teach patients: this is **not for use**
In those with active **chronic flu**.
Use **contraception**—strict and long—
At least **6 months** post-dose is strong.
Black box warning—yes indeed:
For **malignancy** and **fetal need**.

It's **teratogenic**, clear as day,
So pregnancy's a no-go way.
Drug interactions? Immune ones most—
Avoid **live vaccines**, they'll host
Infection risk that spreads too fast—
Wait till immunosuppression's passed.
So **Cladribine**, both sharp and sleek,
Gives long-term calm in just a week.
But guide with labs and patient trust,
For safety first—because it must.

DIMETHYL FUMARATE (TECFIDERA)

Immunomodulator / MS Agent

When **MS flares** and nerves inflame,
Dimethyl Fumarate joins the game.
It shifts immune cells off their track,
To **limit damage and push disease back**.
It **activates Nrf2** in the cell,
A pathway that defends quite well.
With **anti-inflammatory** style,
It shields the brain and slows the trial.
Used for **relapsing forms of MS**,
It helps reduce the flare-up mess.
Not a cure—but it delays
The damage done on rougher days.
Side effects to watch and know:
Flushing, itching, GI blow—
Like **nausea, cramps**, and **diarrhea**,
Especially in that first-dose era.
More serious? Yes—**lymphocytes fall**,
Which can leave them prone to all.
So **PML** (a rare brain threat),
Can occur—don't forget.
Monitor CBCs throughout the year,
Especially as **WBCs disappear**.
Also **LFTs**, keep liver checked,
And signs of infection—always detect.
Teach patients: **take it with food**,
To lessen flushing or upset mood.
Don't crush the capsule, swallow whole,
And stick to schedule as a goal.
No black box warning, but don't dismiss
The **infection risks** that come with this.
And be alert for sudden brain change—
PML can feel quite strange.
Drug interactions? Very few,
But **live vaccines**? Skip that queue.
And avoid **strong immunosuppressants**, too—
Too much suppression won't serve you.
So **Tecfidera**, MS friend,
Helps disease slow—not transcend.
But with labs and careful prep,
It keeps the fire from taking the step.

FINGOLIMOD (GILENYA)
S1P Receptor Modulator / MS Disease-Modifying Agent

When **MS attacks** the nerves again,
And weakness spreads through arm and pen,
Fingolimod slows that decay,
By **locking lymphocytes away**.
It's an **S1P receptor modulator**,
A cell traffic **regulator**.
It traps the T-cells in their base,
So fewer reach the **CNS space**.

Used for **relapsing forms of MS**,
It helps reduce the flare-up mess.
It doesn't cure, but holds the line—
And slows the loss of strength and spine.
Side effects? You must be wise:
Bradycardia, blurred-out eyes.
Headache, fatigue, and **cough** may come,
And **infections** creep when white counts numb.

More rare but real: **macular edema**,
So check the **eyes** for fluid schema.
Liver injury, PML,
And **skin cancer risk** as well.
Monitor before the very first dose—
Do **EKG** and **CBC** close.
Then **observe for 6 hours straight**,
As heart may slow, then modulate.

Check **LFTs**, and test for **zoster** past,
If no vaccine? Then one should be cast.

Also screen for **macular sight**,
And watch for **respiratory** blight.
Teach patients it **modulates immune**,
So avoid the **live vaccines** too soon.
Tell them to report **vision change**,
Or signs of **infection** that feel strange.

Black box warning? Not quite here,
But **serious risks** should still feel near.
Especially with **cardiac disease**,
The first dose could make pulses freeze.
Drug interactions? Take some care—
With **antiarrhythmics**, beware.
And don't combine with **other S1Ps**,
Or overly suppressed immunity creeps.

So **Fingolimod**, MS friend,
Can help the **relapses** suspend.
But given with a watchful hand,
It helps more people **firmly stand**.

GLATIRAMER ACETATE (COPAXONE)

Immunomodulator / MS Disease-Modifying Agent

When **MS flares** and nerves inflame,
And **myelin** breaks in loss and shame,
Glatiramer Acetate stands near—
To **shield the sheath** and make things clear.
A mix of **amino acids four**,
It mimics **myelin** at the core.
This **decoy target** shifts the war,
So **T-cells** fight the drug, not more.

It **modulates the immune response**,
Promotes **Th2 cells** to take the front.
Anti-inflammatory peace it brings,
To help reduce those **MS stings**.
Used for **relapsing MS**, not cure,
But slows progression, firm and pure.
Given **subQ**, it's shot with care—
In **abdomen, arm**, or **thigh spot** there.

Side effects? A modest list:
Injection site lumps, swelling twist.
Flushing, palpitations, chest tight heat,
A brief reaction that's **not repeat**.
No need to **pre-medicate** the scare—
Just let them know it may be there.
Usually it fades away,
In just a few minutes of the day.

Monitor for lipoatrophy's track—
Those **dents in skin** may not bounce back.
Rotate sites to keep things fair,
And use good technique with every care.
Teach patients how to dose at home,
To store it right, not let it roam.
No shaking, freezing, heat, or light—
Just fridge or room temp stored just right.

No black box warning, which is rare,
And **no need for lab draws** in your care.
It's **well-tolerated**, often first,
When other meds may quench or burst.
Drug interactions? Pretty clean—
It doesn't ride the **CYP machine**.
So other meds can stay in place,
No juggling with this MS grace.

So **Copaxone**, safe and tried,
Brings MS warriors steady stride.
With proper teaching, shots, and trust,
It calms the fire without much fuss.

INTERFERON BETA-1A (AVONEX, REBIF)

Immunomodulator / MS Disease-Modifying Agent

When **MS flares** begin to rise,
And **relapses come in fierce disguise**,
Interferon Beta-1a stands tall,
To **slow the damage** and **soften the fall**.
It's an **immunomodulating friend**,
That tells the T-cells: **"Don't descend."**
It calms the **inflammatory drive**,
So nerves and myelin might survive.
Used in **relapsing forms of MS**,
To reduce attacks and daily stress.
It doesn't cure, but still delays
Progression in subtle, steady ways.
Avonex is **once a week IM**,
While **Rebif** gives **subQ** doses again.
Same drug, new rhythm, patient style—
Both meant to help **MS reconcile**.
Side effects? They often bring
A **flu-like feel** with **aching sting**.
Fever, chills, fatigue, myalgia,
Especially in the first-dose saga.
Also watch the **liver strain**,
And signs of **mood shifts**, even pain.
Depression, suicide ideation—
So screen for mental complication.
Monitor: CBCs, LFTs on file,
And **thyroid labs** once in a while.
Watch for **injection site** red or sore,
Especially with Rebif—maybe more.

Teach patients: **premedicate** for chills,
Acetaminophen helps with the ills.
Store it **cold**, and don't forget
To **rotate sites** to prevent regret.
No black box warning, but take care,
Especially with **mood shifts** in the air.
And be alert to **autoimmune signs**,
Like **lupus, thyroid**, or other lines.
Drug interactions? Nothing bold,
But monitor if other **immunosuppressants** are told.
They can **increase infection** risk,
So balance carefully, not brisk.
So **Interferon**, with thoughtful grace,
Helps slow MS in its rough race.

INTERFERON BETA-1B (BETASERON)
Immunomodulator / MS Disease-Modifying Agent

When **myelin frays** and nerves misfire,
And **MS flares** start climbing higher,
Interferon Beta-1b takes aim—
To **calm the storm** and **slow the flame**.
It's an **immunomodulator** strong,
That tells **T-cells** they're in the wrong.
It shifts the body's fierce attack,
To help the **CNS fight back**.
Used for **relapsing MS** defense,
It helps reduce the **flare-up frequency** and **intense**.
Though not a cure, it holds the line,
And gives the nerves a bit more time.
It's **subQ every other day**,
A steady rhythm, dose by day.
Patients learn to self-inject,
With care and timing to protect.
Side effects? A known crew:
Flu-like symptoms—yes, those too.
Chills, fever, aches, and sometimes more,
Especially early—premed helps restore.
Also risk of **liver strain**,
So **LFT monitoring** should remain.
Leukopenia, anemia, too—
So check the **CBC** right through.
Injection site reactions rise—
With **redness, pain**, or **swollen size**.
Rare but serious: mood decline,
So **suicidal thoughts** must stay in line.

Teach patients how to **rotate sites**,
And pre-dose with **NSAIDs** on first nights.
Let them know the chills will fade,
As tolerance builds with each cascade.
No black box warning, yet still smart
To watch for changes in the heart—
Autoimmune risks can come in waves,
So screen for thyroids the body braves.
Drug interactions? Few and light,
But with other **immunosuppressants**, hold tight.
Too much suppression dulls the guard,
And makes infection hit real hard.
So **Betaseron**, bold and clear,
Helps hold back MS's sneer.

MITOXANTRONE (NOVANTRONE)

Immunosuppressant - Rare MS Therapy, Cardiotoxic Risk

A drug once used with hope and drive, To help keep **aggressive MS** alive. **Mitoxantrone** — an old defense, But now it comes with consequence.
An **immunosuppressant**, strong and deep, It makes the **immune attacks** go sleep. It slows down **T-cells**, **B-cells** too, And halts the damage they can do.
Approved for **secondary-progressive**, Or **relapsing MS** that's aggressive. Also used in **cancer care**, But neuro use is now quite rare.
It's given **IV**, not by the mouth, In hospital or clinic route. Every **three months** it's infused, While **cardiac risks** are closely perused.
Cumulative dose is capped and clear— When it's too high, you must veer. Beyond **140 mg/m²**, **Cardiotoxicity** becomes the cost to bear.
Monitor with **echo scans** each time, And watch that **ejection fraction** line. Heart failure signs must be caught, Or damage could be deeply wrought.
It may suppress the **bone marrow**, Causing **neutropenia** in its shadow. So check **WBCs** before each round, Or infections may come unbound.
Blue-green urine might appear, And **amenorrhea** may draw near.

Hair loss, nausea, mouth sores, too— This med has burdens to walk through.
Secondary leukemias may rise, Another risk to recognize. So long-term plans must weigh the gain, Against potential deeper pain.
Never give in **hepatic loss**, Or **cardiac disease** — too high the cost. And pregnancy? A solid "no," Teratogenic risks will grow.
Given all that it can do, Why use this drug? It's strong and true. For those with **worsening MS fast**, When safer meds have long been passed.
But now it's rare, and rightly so— Newer meds have claimed the show. Yet **Mitoxantrone** still holds a place, In textbooks, trials, and cautious grace.

NATALIZUMAB (TYSABRI)
Monoclonal Antibody / Immunomodulator / MS & Crohn's Disease Agent

When **MS flares** don't yield to fight,
And **relapses** strike with all their might,
Natalizumab takes the lead—
To block the cells that cause the bleed.
It's a **monoclonal antibody** true,
Against **α4-integrin's** sticky glue.
It keeps **T-cells** from crossing tight
Into the brain's protective site.

Used for **relapsing MS cases**,
When other drugs have left few traces.
Also helps in **Crohn's disease**,
To calm the gut and bring some ease.
But here's the part that gives us pause:
A rare but serious **immune flaw**.
PML—a brain infection dread,
Can leave the patient **numb or dead**.

So there's a **black box warning** here:
Progressive multifocal leukoencephalopathy—clear.
Caused by **JC virus** gone unbound,
So **screen and monitor** all around.
Side effects beyond that core?
Headache, fatigue, and **joint pain** sore.
Respiratory tract infections too,
And **GI upset** can come through.

Monitor: routine **MRI scans**,
And **neuro checks** with patient plans.
Antibody testing if the risk climbs,
And **liver function** at regular times.
Teach patients the PML signs:
Vision loss, **weakness**, or crossed lines.
Behavior change, or **speech that fails**—
All must prompt fast clinical trails.

It's given **IV once every month**,
In specialty centers, full and blunt.
Because of risk, there's no at-home play—
This med demands a **structured stay**.
Drug interactions? Not a ton,
But avoid with **other immune mods** run.
Stacking suppression raises the score
For PML and danger more.

So **Tysabri**, strong and rare,
Brings hope for those in tough repair.
But only with the greatest care—
Because its risk is always there.

OCRELIZUMAB (OCREVUS)

Monoclonal Antibody / CD20-Directed Cytolytic Agent / MS Disease-Modifying Therapy

When **MS rages** deep inside,
And **nerve insulation** starts to slide,
Ocrelizumab stands tall and bold—
To **calm the flares** and **slow the hold**.
A **monoclonal antibody**, clean,
It targets **CD20's** scene.
Found on **B cells**, young and sly—
It wipes them out before they fly.
Used for **relapsing forms**, for sure,
But also for **PPMS**—a rarer cure.
It's the first that's FDA-cleared
For **progressive MS** long revered.
Side effects you must discuss:
Infusion reactions come with fuss—
Fever, **rash**, **chills**, or even tight chest,
Especially with that **very first test**.
Also risk of **infections high**,
Like **UTIs**, or **respiratory** sigh.
Herpes reactivation too,
So watch for shingles breaking through.
Monitor before infusion day:
Check **hep B**, and clear the way.
Watch **WBC**, and screen with heart,
For signs of cancer that could start.
Black box warning? Not in name,
But **PML** still stakes a claim.
That **JC virus** can sneak in,
So track for **neuro signs** that spin.
Teach patients what to expect:
A **twice-yearly IV** connect.
Premeds help the **reactions dull**,
Like **antihistamines** and steroids full.

Drug interactions? None too known—
It's not a **CYP enzyme** zone.
But avoid live vaccines in flow—
Immune suppression makes them grow.
So **Ocrevus**, with targeted grace,
Slows **MS** in its silent race.
A modern weapon, strong and wise,
To guard the nerves and clear the skies.

OFATUMUMAB (KESIMPTA)

Monoclonal Antibody / CD20-Directed Cytolytic Agent / MS Disease-Modifying Therapy

When **MS attacks** without a break,
And **myelin loss** is hard to take,
Ofatumumab joins the line—
A **B-cell buster**, sleek by design.
It targets **CD20's mark**,
On **B lymphocytes** that fan the spark.
It clears them out with pinpoint aim,
To cool **inflammation** and tame the flame.
Approved for **relapsing MS** kind,
It works to **quiet the immune grind**.
A **monthly shot** you give at home,
So **infusion centers**—leave them alone.
Side effects? A modest list:
Injection site pain, a common twist.
Headache, fever, or **UTI**,
And **nasopharyngitis** passing by.
More rarely still, the **PML fear**,
That **JC virus** lurking near.
So teach the signs that must be tracked—
Vision loss, weakness, focus cracked.
Monitor labs before you start:
Hep B screening plays a part.
CBC, and **immune checks** too,
To watch what B cells try to do.
Teach patients: first doses come
Week 0, 1, 2, then 4—and done!
Then just **once a month** thereafter,
A tiny poke, not IV's chapter.

No black box warning, but stay wise—
Immunosuppression can compromise.
Live vaccines? Those are a no—
Their safety drops when B cells go.
Drug interactions? Few, if any—
It's not in the **CYP mix** like many.
But keep an eye on infection signs,
Especially in crowded lines.
So **Kesimpta**, calm and sharp and neat,
Helps MS warriors **stay on their feet**.
With monthly care and close watch kept,
It slows the damage where it crept.

OZANIMOD (ZEPOSIA)
S1P Receptor Modulator / MS & Ulcerative Colitis Agent

When **immune cells roam** and start to harm,
And **MS flares** bring leg and arm alarm,
Ozanimod steps in the way—
To **trap the T-cells** day by day.
It **modulates S1P receptors**, two:
$S1P_1$ and $S1P_5$ in view.
By locking lymphocytes in nodes,
It keeps them off the CNS roads.

Used for **relapsing MS** today,
And **ulcerative colitis** in the fray.
It tames inflammation's spreading fire,
With daily dosing to inspire.
Side effects? Some may find:
Bradycardia, especially at first time.
Headache, fatigue, nasopharyngitis,
And sometimes **liver enzymes** in crisis.

More serious? **Macular edema**,
So check the eyes—retina schema.
Infections too, and **PML**,
So **monitor closely**, and screen well.
Monitor: EKG pre-first dose,
Especially if heart risk shows.
Do **liver tests**, and check **CBC**,
And test for **VZV immunity**.

Start with **dose titration** slow,
To help the **heart rate** adjust and flow.

Then **once daily** becomes the norm—
With or without food it performs.
Teach patients: no live vaccines,
Until the immune fog routine clears the scene.
And don't stop suddenly on your own,
Or **rebound MS** might be shown.

No black box warning, but still be wise,
About **infection risks** that may arise.
And **macular checks** before you start,
To guard the brain and shield the heart.
Drug interactions? A few to screen:
Avoid **CYP2C8 inhibitors** in between.
And other **immunosuppressants**?
Stacking them brings more consequence.

So **Zeposia**, calm and slick,
Helps **MS symptoms fade and tick**.
A daily pill with guided care,
To slow disease and keep life fair.

PEGINTERFERON BETA-1A (PLEGRIDY)

Immunomodulator / Pegylated Interferon / MS Disease-Modifying Therapy

When **MS relapses** start to rise,
And flare-ups hit like sharp surprise,
Plegridy enters, slow and strong,
To help the flares stay **far and long**.
It's **interferon beta-1a**,
But **pegylated** in its way.
The **PEG chain** makes it last much more—
Just **twice a month**, instead of four.
It's used for **relapsing MS types**,
To **lower flares** and **slow down gripes**.
It tweaks the **immune response** with grace,
And helps inflammation know its place.
Side effects may come in waves:
Flu-like symptoms, muscle raves.
Headache, fever, chills that bite,
And **injection site** reactions bright.
Rare but watchful things include:
Liver issues, shifts in mood.
Suicidal thoughts may grow—
So **monitor mental health** below.
Monitor: CBC, LFT,
And **thyroid labs** routinely.
Check for **depression**, watch them close,
And track for **autoimmune dose**.
Teach patients how to self-inject,
Every 14 days, direct.
Rotate sites and use with care—
And premedicate if flu's still there.
No black box warning, but don't dismiss
That **serious events** can still exist.
PML's a rare and distant fear,
But still, we keep the risk quite clear.

Drug interactions? Not a crowd—
It doesn't touch the CYPs out loud.
But stack with caution if immune
Is being hit from every tune.
So **Plegridy**, with PEG's long tail,
Helps **relapse rates** begin to pale.
A modern twist on interferon's name—
With half the shots, but just the same.

PONESIMOD (PONVORY)
S1P Receptor Modulator / MS Disease-Modifying Therapy

When **MS flares** return once more,
And **T-cells march** to wage their war,
Ponesimod steps in the lane,
To **hold immune cells back** again.
It targets **S1P₁**, just one key—
To **trap lymphocytes** where they should be.
By locking them in lymph node space,
It **slows the flares**, protects the pace.
Used for **relapsing MS disease**,
It helps the brain and spine find ease.
A **daily pill**, well-tolerated,
With **shorter half-life**, calibrated.
Side effects you might expect:
Headache, nausea, chest feels tight at first check.
Liver enzyme bumps, and **cold-like feels**,
And sometimes **BP softly reels**.
There's risk for **bradycardia**, too—
So watch that **first dose** very true.
First-dose observation may apply,
If **heart history** walks nearby.
Monitor: EKG before you start,
LFTs, CBC, and **eye and heart**.
Check for **macular edema** signs,
And **VZV titers** in patient lines.
Teach patients: titrate slow—
14-day starter pack helps it flow.
Take it **once a day**, the same each time,
And **don't stop suddenly**—that's the line.

No black box warning, but stay aware
Of **infection risks** with lowered care.
Avoid **live vaccines** during play—
Their safety fades in that delay.
Drug interactions? A few for sure:
With **CYP2C9 and 3A4**,
Strong inducers or inhibitors can
Alter levels—adjust the plan.
So **Ponvory**, sleek and small,
Helps **MS warriors** stand tall.
With daily rhythm, labs, and care,
It helps reduce the flares out there.

68

SIPONIMOD (MAYZENT)
S1P Receptor Modulator / MS Disease-Modifying Therapy

When **MS creeps** in quiet disguise,
And **progression starts** behind the eyes,
Siponimod steps up with might—
To hold back loss and slow the fight.
It targets **S1P$_1$ and S1P$_5$**,
To keep **lymphocytes** from taking dives
Into the brain and spinal cord,
Where damage often strikes the board.

Approved for **SPMS** that's active still,
And **relapsing MS** types that spill.
It helps reduce the **annual flares**,
And slows decline with daily care.
But before you start, here's the check:
A **CYP2C9 genotype spec**.
Because metabolism shifts the game—
Some variants **shouldn't dose the same**.

Side effects? A careful lot:
Headache, **hypertension**, vision caught.
Liver enzymes may rise high,
And **bradycardia** can apply.
Macular edema can appear—
So test the **eyes** before you steer.
And watch for **PML**, although rare,
With **JC virus**, stay aware.

Monitor: EKG and **LFT**,
CBC, and **vision**, just to be.

Also check for **infections** near—
The immune system's downshifted gear.
Teach patients: start with **titration slow**,
For 5 to 6 days before you go.
Then it's **once daily**, same time each day,
With or without food, that's okay.

No black box warning, but take note—
Infection, cardiac, all should float.
Live vaccines? Put them on pause—
Your immune defense might miss the cause.
Drug interactions? A few to flag:
With **CYP2C9/CYP3A4**, don't lag.
Avoid strong **modulators** that
Can tip the balance off the mat.

So **Mayzent**, small but tightly keyed,
Helps meet the **progression** MS breeds.
With testing first and slow advance,
It gives the nervous system a chance.

TERIFLUNOMIDE (AUBAGIO)
Pyrimidine Synthesis Inhibitor / MS Disease-Modifying Agent

When **MS flares** begin to rise,
And **relapses catch you by surprise**,
Teriflunomide holds the line—
To **slow the immune system's climb**.
It blocks **dihydroorotate dehydrogenase**,
A mouthful, but it earns its praise.
By halting **pyrimidine's** steady birth,
It stops T-cells from gaining girth.
Used in **relapsing MS forms**,
To **reduce attacks** and **dampen storms**.
A **once-daily pill**, so easy to take,
With **long effects** in each small break.
Side effects? A few to watch:
Hair thinning, **nausea**, and liver blotch.
Headache, **diarrhea**, sometimes fatigue,
And **infections** sneaking through the league.
Black box warning—yes, it's true:
Hepatotoxicity can come through.
So **LFTs** before and during the run,
To catch the risk before it's begun.
Also **teratogenic**, strong and clear—
Not safe for pregnancy anywhere near.
So birth control is **non-negotiable**,
And planning? Fully **discussable**.
Teach patients: long washout plan—
It **sticks around** more than most can.

Cholestyramine or **activated charcoal**
Helps flush it from the body's hold.
Monitor: CBC, LFTs on file,
And blood pressure every once in a while.
And test for **TB** before you start—
A latent case could play its part.
Drug interactions? Yes, a few:
It's metabolized with **CYP2C8** in view.
So **repaglinide**, **pioglitazone**,
May need a shift in their dose tone.
So **Aubagio**, sleek and small,
Helps **MS patients** stand more tall.
With daily dosing and close watch kept,
It slows the flames where they've long crept.

Part IV
Migraine & CGRP Antagonists

ALMOTRIPTAN (AXERT)
Selective Serotonin (5-HT B/1D) Receptor Agonist - Triptan Class

When **migraine pain** begins to strike,
Almotriptan helps things feel right.
It's a **triptan drug**, a **serotonin friend**,
That makes those pounding headaches end.
It binds **5-HT₁B and D**,
Constricts those vessels, sets pain free.
It stops **neurogenic inflammation**,
Restoring peace to the cranial nation.

Used for **acute migraine** when it hits,
But **not for prevention** or daily blitz.
Best if taken early, fast—
To make the pounding moment pass.
Side effects? Let's list a few:
Dizziness, **sleepiness**, maybe **flu**.
Some feel **numbness**, **tightness**, or **pain**,
In **chest or throat**—that's not so plain.

No-go if there's **cardiac disease**,
Or **stroke** or **HTN that won't ease**.
Avoid in those with **peripheral woes**,
And don't combine with **ergot bros**.
Monitor for pain in chest or head,
And signs that oxygen's underfed.
Look for **serotonin syndrome signs**,
If on **SSRIs**, cross-check lines.

Teach patients not to **take too many**,
Two per day's the upper limit, any
More can cause **rebound pain** to swell,
So track the dose and time it well.
No **black box warning**, but don't forget,
To rule out heart risks—always vet.
And interactions? Watch with care—
SSRIs, **MAOIs**, and **linezolid** beware.

So **Almotriptan**, short and sweet,
Can knock a migraine off its feet.
Used with care, it works just right,
To dim that pounding, blinding light.

ATOGEPANT (QULIPTA)
CGRP Antagonist – Oral Migraine Prevention

To keep the migraines far at bay, **Atogepant** is taken each day. An **oral CGRP block**, it's clear— To stop the storm before it's near.
Unlike the meds for pain in flight, **Qulipta** guards both day and night. It's **preventative**, not rescue care, It works before the pain is there.
It binds to **CGRP receptors tight**, And blocks the signal's flaming light. So trigeminal nerves won't shout, And blood vessel chaos stays out.
Once-daily pill, no shots or sprays, A smooth approach for busy days. It's well-tolerated and quite mild, Approved for adults—not for child.
Nausea, **fatigue**, and **appetite loss**, Are side effects to watch and cross. **Constipation** comes up the most, So fiber fans may need to post.
It's safe for those with cardiac strain, No **vasoconstriction** in the vein. So folks who can't take triptans well, Find **Qulipta** works without the spell.
No need to time it with auras or pain, Just **take it daily** to maintain. It reduces **monthly migraine days**, And lets the mind explore new ways.
Avoid with drugs that **raise its level**, Like **ketoconazole**, a known dishevel. **Liver caution** may apply, So screen before the first supply.
It's not for treating pain that's here— It's for the days you long to clear. Prevention is its only lane, Don't take it when you're deep in pain.

Compare it with its sister meds— Like **Nurtec** or the **Aimovig** threads. Each has its own kind of use, But **Atogepant** keeps the moose loose.
So if the headaches steal your week, And daily joy is hard to seek, **Qulipta** might just be the key— To break the chain and set you free.

DIHYDROERGOTAMINE (MIGRANAL)
Ergot Alkaloid / Antimigraine Agent

When **migraine auras** start to flare,
And pounding pain is hard to bear,
Dihydroergotamine steps in,
To stop the storm before it spins.
An **ergot alkaloid**, sharp and tight,
It **binds serotonin receptors** right.
5-HT,D and 1B, to be exact—
It **vasoconstricts** and stops attack.
Used in **acute migraine events**,
And sometimes for **cluster headaches** intense.
It won't prevent, but treats in time,
When throbbing heads begin to climb.
Side effects can still appear:
Nausea, rhinitis, bitter fear.
Dizziness, tingling, flushing, too,
And **injection site pain** may come through.
More rare but serious—**vasospasm**,
That cuts off flow in heart or chasm.
So don't give if there's **CAD**,
HTN, or **vascular history**.
Black box warning waves its flag:
Don't use with **strong CYP3A4**—it's a drag.
Like **macrolides** or **protease crew**,
They raise the risk of **ischemia**, too.
Monitor for chest pain or signs
Of **poor perfusion** in limbs or minds.
Watch **BP, pulse**, and **neuro vibe**,
Especially if they're older tribe.
Teach patients: **don't use daily**, no—
Limit to **twice a week or so**.
And **nasal spray**? They must be clear
To **prime** the pump and aim it near.
Drug interactions? Quite a few—
Avoid with **triptans, MAOIs**, too.
And **SSRIs** can sometimes share
A **serotonin syndrome** scare.
So **Migranal**, a niche but mighty tool,
Can stop a migraine's spinning rule.
But used with caution, space, and grace—
It keeps the pain from taking place.

ELETRIPTAN (RELPAX)
Selective Serotonin (5-HT B/1D) Receptor Agonist – Triptan Class

When **migraine thunder** starts to grow,
And lights and sounds all start to blow,
Eletriptan comes in to fight,
To **constrict the vessels** and make things right.
A **triptan drug**, it's sharp and fast,
It binds **5-HT,B and 1D** class.
It calms the trigeminal nerve's release,
To bring the pounding pain to peace.
Used for **acute migraine attack**,
But **not for prevention**—don't look back.
Best when taken **at first sign**,
To stop the storm before it climbs.
Side effects may still appear:
Dizziness, fatigue, or **chest pain** near.
Some feel **tingling**, others tight,
In **jaw or neck**, with awkward fright.
Avoid in folks with **heart disease**,
Or **stroke**, **HTN** that won't appease.
It **raises BP** and **shrinks the flow**,
So clogged-up arteries say no.
Monitor for signs of strain,
Like **chest discomfort, tingling brain**.
And always ask if **aura's new**—
Could mean a stroke is peeking through.

Teach patients: one dose first, then pause,
If no relief—**repeat with cause**,
But not more than **two a day**,
And **20 mg** is max okay.
No black box warning, but be smart,
It can affect the **head and heart**.
And wait **24 hours** if switching teams—
Don't mix with **ergots** or **other triptan dreams**
Drug interactions? Yes, indeed:
With **CYP3A4 inhibitors**, slow your speed.
Like **ketoconazole** or **clarithromycin**,
They raise the drug too high within.
So **Relpax** brings the lightning down,
And wipes away that migraine frown.
With proper timing, dose, and check,
It puts that pounding pain in check.

EPTINEZUMAB (VYEPTI)
CGRP Monoclonal Antibody / Migraine Prevention Agent

When **migraines hit** month after month,
And **aura** comes with throbbing punch,
Eptinezumab steps in smooth—
To help the cycles slow and soothe.
It's a **monoclonal antibody**, clean,
That blocks **CGRP** from causing a scene.
Calcitonin Gene-Related Peptide—that's the source,
Of migraine's wild and painful course.

It's used for **prevention**, not attack,
To keep the migraines from coming back.
Given **IV every 3 months or so**,
To keep that daily pressure low.
Side effects are mostly tame:
Nasal congestion, allergy name.
Fatigue, itching, sore throat here,
But serious risks are pretty rare.

Still, watch for signs of **hypersensitivity**,
Like **rash**, **tight chest**, or **swelling rapidly**.
Though anaphylaxis is rare to see,
Monitor post-infusion carefully.
Teach patients it's not for pain that's begun,
But to help reduce how **often** they come.
It won't replace your rescue med—
It just keeps migraine days in check instead.

No black box warning, but always wise
To watch **immune response** that may arise.
It's not yet known if it's safe in all—
Like **pregnant patients**—so proceed with call.
Drug interactions? None well known—
It's not metabolized through CYP enzyme zones.
So far, it plays well in the crowd,
But long-term data's not fully loud.

So **Vyepti**, with its quarterly drip,
Helps chronic migraine lose its grip.
A preventive strike in antibody form,
To keep the brain a little more warm.

ERENUMAB (AIMOVIG)
CGRP Receptor Antagonist / Migraine Prevention Agent

When **migraines** crash your life each week,
And **pain and aura** feel too bleak,
Erenumab steps in with might,
To help reduce that daily fight.
It blocks the **CGRP receptor** clear,
Where **calcitonin peptides** interfere.
By stopping CGRP's painful shout,
It helps keep **vasodilation** out.
Used for **migraine prevention**, bold—
In **episodic** or **chronic** hold.
It's **once-monthly** and given sub-Q,
A shot you or your patient can do.
Side effects are fairly few:
Constipation is the most common clue.
Also **injection site reactions**, slight,
And sometimes **muscle cramps at night**.
Rare but real? **Allergic flares**,
Like **angioedema** or **hives** in pairs.
So if there's swelling in the face,
Seek help fast—just in case.
Monitor for adverse tone,
Especially if they're using it at home.
Track migraine days before and after,
To gauge if life has started to feel lighter.
Teach patients: This won't stop a storm,
But helps prevent the migraine norm.
It might take **a few months** to feel,
The full preventive power it can seal.
No black box warning—none today,
But use with care, the cautious way.
Safety in **pregnancy**? Not yet known,
So best to hold if babies are grown.
Drug interactions? Not a fuss—
Not metabolized through **CYPs** like us.
So no big worries with polypharm,
Which adds to this med's calming charm.
So **Erenumab**, sleek and clean,
Aims to keep the head more serene.
With monthly dose and guided plan,
It gives migraine relief a better span.

FREMANEZUMAB (AJOVY)
CGRP Monoclonal Antibody / Migraine Prevention Agent

When **monthly migraines** cloud the skies,
And every trigger multiplies,
Fremanezumab steps in clean—
To calm the storm before it's seen.
A **monoclonal antibody**, sleek,
It finds **CGRP** and makes it weak.
That peptide's key in **migraine's pain**,
So blocking it can **ease the brain**.
It's used for **prevention**, not attack—
To **keep those headaches from coming back**.
For **chronic** or **episodic** woes,
It helps reduce the migraine blows.
Given subQ, once a month or three,
A flexible **dosing** strategy.
And with a half-life long and wide,
It keeps that CGRP outside.
Side effects? They're mostly few:
Injection site pain, mild and true.
Fatigue, **constipation**, maybe cold,
But serious risks? Rarely told.
Still, watch for **allergic signs**,
Like **swelling**, **rash**, or troubled lines.
Though rare, **hypersensitivity**
Should be managed immediately.
Monitor how migraines behave,
Track the days that it may save.
Remind them: **not for sudden spikes**—
Their **rescue med** still has the likes.
No **black box warning**, but still wise

To check if **CGRP blockers** harmonize.
And though it's safe in most you see,
Its use in **pregnancy** lacks guarantee.
Drug interactions? Not well known—
It doesn't touch **CYP enzyme zone**.
So it plays nice with other meds,
And rarely causes dosing dreads.
So **Ajovy**, calm and clear,
Can make those migraines disappear.
With once-a-month or quarterly aim,
It keeps the head from migraine flame.

FROVATRIPTAN (FROVA)
Selective Serotonin (5-HT B/1D) Receptor Agonist - Triptan Class

When **migraine shadows** start to creep,
And pain comes crashing into sleep,
Frovatriptan brings relief—
A **longer-lasting, migraine thief**.
A **triptan** with a slower start,
It still **constricts those vessels'** part.
It binds to **5-HT,B/1D**,
To stop the throbbing pain cascade.
Best for those with **menstrual strain**,
Whose migraines come with hormone rain.
Its **half-life's long**—a full 26,
So it helps prevent **those rebound tricks**.
Side effects are mostly mild:
Dizziness, fatigue, or pressure wild.
Chest or neck tightness, transient flares,
And sometimes **dry mouth** unawares.
But triptan rules still apply—
Avoid if **cardiac risks** are high.
Stroke, HTN, vascular clogs—
This med is **not for those backlogs**.
Monitor for heart-type signs,
Like **pain that spreads** or weird **spine lines**.
And make sure they know the goal—
It's **not for prevention**, just **pain control**.
Teach patients: **take it at first sign**,
And they may need a **second line**.
But no more than **2 in 24**,
Or side effects may come to the fore.

No black box warning, but don't forget—
It **can't be mixed with ergots** yet.
And wait a day if switching triptans—
Don't stack serotonin like quicksand.
Drug interactions? Just a few—
Be careful with **SSRIs**, too.
And **MAOIs**? That's a no—
Could make the serotonin overflow.
So **Frovatriptan**, steady and strong,
Works best when **migraines linger long**.
With careful timing, dose, and track,
It helps keep migraine monsters back.

GALCANEZUMAB (EMGALITY)

CGRP Monoclonal Antibody / Migraine & Cluster Headache Prevention

When **migraines loom** like storms ahead,
And **cluster pain** brings nightly dread,
Galcanezumab steps in strong,
To **block CGRP** all month long.
A **monoclonal antibody**, sleek,
It **targets CGRP**—the pain-link tweak.
By binding it before it lands,
It helps uncramp those vessel strands.
It's used to **prevent migraine pain**,
And **cluster headaches' brutal chain**.
With **monthly shots**, it works with grace,
To lower **attack days** and keep your pace.
Side effects? A mellow field:
Injection site pain, perhaps not healed.
Some get **itching**, **dizziness**, or feel
Constipation in the deal.
Rarely, **hypersensitivity**
May cause **rash** or **swelling** suddenly.
So teach them signs and when to call,
Especially if symptoms sprawl.
Monitor the **frequency of attacks**,
To see how well the med fights back.
No need to check labs in routine—
But track how well their days stay clean.

Teach patients how to give the shot,
In **abdomen**, **thigh**, or **arm's soft spot**.
It's **once per month**, or **two weeks' pace**
For **clusters** in their active phase.
No black box warning shadows near,
But use with **caution** if risks appear.
Pregnancy safety isn't quite known,
So hold off there or use it shown.
Drug interactions? Minimal mess—
No **CYP pathways**, so not much stress.
It plays well with most migraine stacks,
And doesn't require cutting back.
So **Emgality**, clean and clear,
Helps migraines slowly disappear.
With needle, plan, and monthly guide,
It keeps the pounding storms outside.

LASMIDITAN (REYVOW)
Selective 5-HT F Receptor Agonist / Acute Migraine Agent

When **migraine strikes** without a warn,
And light and sound feel sharp and torn,
Lasmiditan steps in with care,
To ease the pain that pulses there.
It's not a **triptan**—that's the key,
No **vasoconstriction** here, you see.
It targets **5-HT₁F** instead,
To calm the **trigeminal threads**.

Used for **acute migraine pain**,
When nausea, light, and throbs remain.
It's great for those with **cardiac risk**,
Who can't take triptans in their mix.
Side effects? A central kind:
Dizziness, sleepy, slowed-down mind.
Fatigue, numbness, hallucination,
A true **CNS sedation**.

So **monitor** before they drive,
Because reaction time may dive.
It's **Schedule V**—not often seen
For migraine meds, but fits this scene.
Teach patients: **take at onset fast**,
But **one dose only**—make it last.
No second try within a day—
It's **one and done**, then pain delay.

No black box warning, but be wise:
This drug affects **alertness** ties.
And **serotonin syndrome** might arise,
With **SSRIs or SNRIs**.
Drug interactions? Yes, a few—
Other CNS depressants, too.
And **CYP3A4 inhibitors** might
Change the levels—track them right.

So **Reyvow**, new and triptan-free,
Brings relief to those with **cardiac history**.
A non-constricting pain control,
To help the migraine lose its hold.

NARATRIPTAN (AMERGE)
Selective 5-HT B/1D Receptor Agonist / Antimigraine Agent

When **migraines creep** with subtle start,
And drill their ache into your heart,
Naratriptan brings relief—
A **triptan** choice that's calm and brief.
It binds to **5-HT₁B and 1D**,
To **constrict the vessels** clean.
It tames the **trigeminal nerve's release**,
And helps the migraine **fade in peace**.
Used for **mild-to-moderate attack**,
With **longer half-life**, holding back.
It's **slower onset**, but with grace—
Less likely to cause **rebound chase**.
Side effects may still arise:
Tingling, warmth, or **dizzy skies**.
Chest pressure, fatigue, or pain,
Though usually they're **mild and plain**.
Not for those with heart disease,
Or **stroke, hypertension**, histories.
Because it **constricts** the arteries tight,
And could cause **ischemic fright**.
Monitor for aura strange,
Or neuro signs that start to change.
Teach patients: take it at first sign,
Then wait **four hours** before next line.
Max dose? Two tabs per day—
Beyond that, side effects may play.
And **not for prevention**, just attack—
So don't use daily to push pain back.

No black box warning, but take care,
With **serotonergic meds** out there.
Serotonin syndrome, though rare,
Can sneak up with that combo flare.
Drug interactions? A few in scope:
MAOIs? A definite nope.
Wait **24 hours** between triptan teams,
And avoid with **ergotamine dreams**.
So **Naratriptan**, mild and long,
Works best for migraines **not too strong**.
It's gentle, steady, thoughtfully made—
A softer triptan that holds its grade.

RIZATRIPTAN (MAXALT)
Selective 5-HT B/1D Receptor Agonist / Antimigraine Agent

When **migraine pain** begins to roar,
And light and noise you can't ignore,
Rizatriptan comes fast and tight—
To **close the vessels**, block the fight.
It's a **5-HT,B/1D**
Receptor agonist, sharp and clean.
It **constricts the cranial flow**,
And stops the neuropeptides' show.
Used for **acute migraine attacks**,
With or without **aura tracks**.
It's not for daily use or guard—
Just when the pain is coming hard.
Maxalt melts or swallows whole—
ODT or tablet meets the goal.
Relief can come in **30 minutes'** time,
So take it early in the climb.
Side effects? A triptan crew:
Chest pressure, tightness, tingling, too.
Drowsiness, dizziness, jaw or neck pain,
And sometimes **dry mouth** may remain.
**Not for use in heart disease,
Stroke, uncontrolled BP**, or if **vessels seize**.
Because it **constricts**, it's not for all—
Screen history well before you call.

Teach patients: take **at first sign**,
A second dose is **allowed in time**—
But **wait 2 hours**, and **no more than 30 mg a day**,
Or side effects may find their way.
No black box warning, but beware
Of **serotonin syndrome** with meds out there.
Like **SSRIs, SNRIs** too—
Stacking them can harm you through.
Drug interactions? Yes, take note:
Propranolol affects this boat.
If combined, the dose should shrink—
The levels rise more than you think.
So **Maxalt**, quick and clinically slick,
Can **kick a migraine** out real quick.
But always used with mindful care—
For vessels, mood, and meds out there.

RIMEGEPANT (NURTEC ODT)

CGRP Receptor Antagonist / Acute & Preventive Migraine Agent

When **migraine pain** begins to grow,
And pounding temples steal your flow,
Rimegepant dissolves with speed—
To meet both **acute** and **preventive** need.
It blocks the **CGRP receptor's gate**,
To stop that neuropeptide fate.
No vasoconstriction in its route—
Just **calm the chaos**, ease the bout.

Used to treat a **migraine attack**,
Or take it **every other day** to keep them back.
One pill that **melts beneath the tongue**,
A **dual-use med**, both sharp and young.
Side effects? They're mostly few:
Nausea, fatigue, and tummy flu.
Some feel **dry mouth**, or get a **rash**,
But most get by without a clash.

No risk of **rebound pain rebound**,
So **daily triptans** can be unbound.
Safe in folks with **heart disease**,
Which triptans don't permit with ease.
Monitor for signs of rare—
Hypersensitivity in the air.

Rash, trouble breathing, swelling face—
Stop and seek a safer space.

Teach patients: for **acute**, take one,
No more in **24 hours** done.
For **prevention**, every other day—
With water, no food in the way.
No black box warning, which is sweet,
But still watch for **drug interactions** in the sheet.
CYP3A4—it rides that line,
So avoid with grapefruit or ketoconazole's shine.

So **Nurtec**, light and cherry-slick,
Brings **CGRP relief real quick**.
A migraine fighter, modern, clean—
For rescue or for keeping lean.

SUMATRIPTAN (IMITREX)
Selective 5-HT B/1D Receptor Agonist / Antimigraine Agent

When **migraine strikes** and pulses pound,
And light and noise spin all around,
Sumatriptan hits the track—
To bring your **clarity** right back.
It binds to **5-HT,B and 1D**,
To **constrict the vessels** clean.
It also stops **CGRP's release**,
To **calm the nerves** and bring you peace.
Used for **acute migraine attacks**,
It doesn't stop them from coming back.
But taken **early**, it can slay
The pain that tries to wreck your day.
Forms? You've got quite a spread—
Tablet, nasal, auto-inject instead.
The **subQ shot** acts fastest yet,
For pain that's peaking like a threat.
Side effects? The triptan crew:
Tingling, chest tightness, flushing too.
Drowsiness, jaw or throat feels strange,
But usually brief and within range.
Contraindicated in hearts not strong—
CAD, stroke, or **HTN gone wrong**.
Since it **constricts blood vessels**, be wise—
Not for those with **vascular compromise**.
Teach patients: take it **right at the start**,
And wait **2 hours** if second parts.

Max dose? Just **200 mg per day**,
Depending on the route and way.
No black box warning, but take heed
Of **serotonin syndrome**, especially when you lead
With **SSRIs, SNRIs** near—
Too much serotonin's a thing to fear.
Drug interactions? Yes, be alert:
MAOIs will make it hurt.
Avoid **ergots** within 24,
And watch your **CNS med** drawer.
So **Imitrex**, the OG triptan,
Works fast and firm with a solid plan.
For migraines sharp, and aura bright,
It brings the calm back into sight.

UBROGEPANT (UBRELVY)
CGRP Receptor Antagonist / Acute Migraine Agent

When **migraine strikes** without a sound,
And **pounding pressure** starts to mount,
Ubrogepant steps in fast—
To help the **storm inside you pass**.
It blocks the **CGRP receptor** gates,
To ease the pain that **neuropeptide** creates.
No vessel squeeze like triptans do—
Just targets where the peptides flew.

Used to treat **migraine acute**,
When light and sound are hard to mute.
But not for daily **prevention's lane**—
Just when the **throbbing** starts again.
Side effects? A minor stack:
Nausea, **dry mouth**, **sleepy track**.
Some feel **fatigue**, or stomach strain,
But serious risks are fairly plain.

No black box warning, and no fear
Of **vasoconstriction** lurking near.
So it's safe for those whose **hearts can't take**
The **triptan route** for migraine ache.
Teach patients: take **one at onset**,
Then **wait two hours** if pain's not gone yet.
A **second dose** can sometimes help—
But **200 mg max daily** for yourself.

Drug interactions? Yep, a few:
CYP3A4 inhibitors skew
The levels higher—so reduce the dose
When meds like **ketoconazole** are close.
No need to avoid foods or light,
Just keep it close for migraine fight.
It works best when it's taken early—
Right as the pain begins to curl-y.

So **Ubrelvy**, modern, safe, and clean,
Brings migraine warriors back serene.
With gentle touch and peptide block,
It stops the tick of migraine's clock.

ZOLMITRIPTAN (ZOMIG)
Selective 5-HT B/1D Receptor Agonist / Antimigraine Agent

When **aura flashes** and throbbing starts,
And migraines tear your day apart,
Zolmitriptan comes swift and clean—
To stop the surge **unseen, routine**.
It binds to **5-HT,B and 1D**,
To **constrict cranial vessels** clean.
And blocks the **CGRP release**,
To bring the pounding brain some peace.
Used for **acute migraine attack**,
With or without **aura's track**.
It **won't prevent**—just stop the pain,
When headaches start to roar again.
Zomig comes in **three strong forms**:
Tablet, ODT, and **nasal storms**.
The **nasal spray** works fast and fine,
For migraines in their rapid climb.
Side effects? Like triptans do:
Tingling, tightness, pressure, too.
Drowsiness, dry mouth, flushing face,
And sometimes **weird sensations** race.
Not for those with **heart disease**,
Stroke, or **uncontrolled BP**.
It **constricts the vessels**, so beware—
In vascular risk, don't go there.
Teach patients: take it **early on**,
When migraine signs have just begun.
One dose now, then wait two hours—
A second dose is in your powers.
Max dose? It holds the line—
10 mg per day, you'll be fine.
And **no more than two doses** through,
To keep side effects far from you.
No black box warning, but take care
With **serotonin meds** out there.
Serotonin syndrome is rare,
But worth a pause and patient stare.
Drug interactions? CYPs apply—
1A2 inhibitors amplify.
Cimetidine, for one, may raise
Its levels in unexpected ways.
So **Zomig**, sleek and ready-made,
Helps **migraine misery** start to fade.

ZAVEGEPANT (ZAVZPRET)
CGRP Antagonist - Nasal Migraine Rescue

A migraine strikes with blinding might, The world too loud, the room too bright. But **Zavegepant**, a nasal spray, Can help that pain to fade away.

A **CGRP receptor blocker** true, It stops the peptide breaking through. No **vasodilation**, no more flame— It interrupts the migraine game.

It's used as **acute migraine aid**, When nausea or pills invade. **One spray per nostril**—that's the rule, To beat the pain and keep things cool.

Zavzpret works within **two hours**, Restoring strength and quiet powers. And unlike triptans, it's allowed When heart disease has been avowed.

It's **not a preventative med**, But taken when the pain is spread. For those who suffer once or more, This **nasal route** can help restore.

Side effects are mostly tame: **Taste disorder** leads the blame. **Nausea, throat pain**, maybe sneeze— But far less than a triptan tease.

No **vasoconstriction** here, So safer in those hearts we fear. That makes it helpful far and wide, Where others can't be safely tried.

Don't mix with **CYP3A4 strong**, Like **ketoconazole** — that goes wrong. No need for dose to escalate, One puff is all you regulate.

It's brand new, just approved in time, With fast results and dosing prime. **Zavegepant** joins CGRP's team, To offer patients a new dream.

Nurtec, **Ubrelvy** came before, But this is **nasal**, not a chore. A breakthrough for those who can't wait, Or vomit pills they try to take. So when the migraine knocks you down, And nothing helps but staying bound, Try **Zavegepant**, quick and clean— A nasal mist for pain unseen.

Part V
Alzheimer's, Dementia & Cognitive Decline

DONEPEZIL (ARICEPT)
Cholinesterase Inhibitor / Alzheimer's Agent

When **memory fades** and thoughts grow thin,
And **Alzheimer's** slowly creeps within,
Donepezil lends some aid,
To **keep the mind from quick degrade**.
It **blocks acetylcholinesterase**,
So **ACh** can stick around and blaze.
This helps with **cognition**, mood, and flow,
Though **progression** still may go.
Used for **mild to severe dementia**, yes—
In **Alzheimer's**, it's one of the best.
It doesn't cure, but slows the slide,
And brings back clarity for a ride.
Side effects you need to note:
Nausea, **vomiting**, GI bloat.
Bradycardia, **fainting**, too,
And **insomnia** may break through.
Rare but serious? **Rhabdomyolysis**,
And **seizures**—though these are hit-or-miss.
GI bleeds and **heart block** can unfold,
Especially in patients **frail or old**.
Monitor for HR dropping low,
And **GI signs** that start to grow.
Also watch for **weight and mood**,
And if they're eating enough food.
Teach patients: **take at bedtime** first,
To lessen nausea at its worst.
And **don't stop suddenly**—taper slow,
So the system won't misfire or go.

No black box warning, but keep alert,
The **cardiac risks** can still hurt.
Use caution in those with **asthma**, too,
As more ACh may tighten through.
Drug interactions? Several, yes—
With **anticholinergics**, it's a mess.
Avoid things that blunt ACh's flow,
Or the med's effects may never show.
So **Donepezil**, with gentle aim,
Helps preserve the **cognitive flame**.
A slowing tool for time and grace,
To help them hold a name, a face.

GALANTAMINE (RAZADYNE, RAZADYNE ER)

Acetylcholinesterase Inhibitor / Alzheimer's Agent

When **memories fade** and thoughts grow thin,
And **Alzheimer's** starts creeping in,
Galantamine lends its grace,
To help the mind hold time and place.
It **blocks acetylcholinesterase**,
So **ACh** stays to light the maze.
But that's not all—it boosts the flame
At **nicotinic receptors**, earning fame.
Used for **mild to moderate decline**,
It helps preserve **function over time**.
Not a cure, but slows the fall,
And helps recall a name, a call.
Side effects may tag along:
Nausea, **vomiting**, not too strong.
Bradycardia, **fainting**, GI pains,
Insomnia, **weight loss**, or **urine strains**.
Rare but real: **skin reactions** dire—
Like **Stevens-Johnson's blistered fire**.
So if there's **rash** that spreads or burns,
Stop the med—don't wait turns.
Monitor weight and mental state,
Track **HR** and **GI fate**.
And if they're frail or prone to fall,
Adjust the dose or pause the call.
Teach patients: **take with food**, not bare,
To soften stomach's quick despair.
Start low, go slow, with titration care,
And don't stop fast—it's not a dare.
No black box warning, but still wise
To check for **cardiac compromise**.
And avoid in those who can't sustain
A **drop in heart rate** through the brain.
Drug interactions? Yes, a few—
With **anticholinergics**, it won't do.
They cancel each other, dull the shine—
So pick one side of the cholinergic line.
So **Galantamine**, gentle and bright,
Helps keep the brain within the light.
With careful watch and dosing plan,
It slows the drift where minds began.

MEMANTINE (NAMENDA)
NMDA Receptor Antagonist / Alzheimer's Disease Agent

When **memories fade** and minds retreat,
And **Alzheimer's** makes time incomplete,
Memantine steps in, calm and slow,
To **ease the noise where signals flow**.
It blocks the **NMDA gate**,
Where **glutamate** can overstate.
By dampening this constant stream,
It gives the brain a bit more gleam.
Used for **moderate to severe decline**,
In **dementia's** later, foggier time.
It won't restore what's gone away,
But may help **clarity** stay at bay.
Often paired with **AChE meds**,
Like **Donepezil**, as science treads.
Together they may help extend
Cognition just a little bend.
Side effects? A modest crew:
Dizziness, headache, maybe flu.
Constipation, hallucination,
And rarely, mood's **agitation**.
Monitor mental tone and mood,
And check for changes that intrude.
Also screen for **renal strain**,
As dose adjusts with **kidney pain**.
Teach patients: titrate slow,
Start with **5 mg**, then up we go.
It's taken once or twice a day—
With or without food—either way.
No black box warning, but still wise
To keep a watchful set of eyes.
Confusion, falls, or **urine flow**
Should all be tracked as symptoms grow.

Drug interactions? Mostly tame—
But avoid with **other NMDA** in name.
And use care with **alkaline urine**,
It can affect how drug levels begin.
So **Memantine**, gentle, firm, and kind,
Helps quiet down the cluttered mind.
A thoughtful ally in the race
To slow dementia's forward pace.

METHYLPHENIDATE PATCH (DAYTRANA)

Stimulant – Transdermal ADHD & Cognitive Support (Off-Label)

A patch that fuels the focus game, **Daytrana** is its branded name. A **methylphenidate** release, To help the mind regain its peace.
Approved for **ADHD** in youth, It helps with focus, speed, and truth. But sometimes used off-label wide, To **boost cognition** on the side.
The patch goes on the **hip each day**, Where meds absorb in gentle sway. A **transdermal stimulant**, rare to see, That offers kids and teens some ease.
Blocks reuptake of dopamine, And **norepinephrine**, so it's clean. It sharpens thoughts, improves the drive, To keep the frontal lobes alive.
Applied in morning, lasts all day, But **pull it off** if side effects stay.
Two hours to kick — so plan with care, And dose remains for hours there.
Insomnia, **appetite decline**, Are side effects that show in line.
Irritability, **racing heart**, Or **tics** may rise — so play it smart.
It's **Schedule II**, a drug controlled, Abuse potential must be told. So lock it up, and sign it out, Each patch accounted, there's no doubt. Rotate the site to save the skin, And press for seconds to begin. Don't cut or heat or alter form— It breaks the seal and harms the norm.
Not used in kids **under six years**, And monitor for growth arrears.
Height and weight each visit track, To catch delays and help bounce back.
In adults, it's used at times For **TBI** or **off-label climbs**. In elders too, it's tried discreet When **memory loss** becomes concrete.
Yet patches must be handled well, And patients taught so all goes swell. **Daytrana's path** is smooth but strong— For those who need their focus long.

RIVASTIGMINE (EXELON)
Acetylcholinesterase Inhibitor / Alzheimer's & Parkinson's Dementia Agent

When **memories fade** and thoughts decline,
And time slips by without a sign,
Rivastigmine steps in slow—
To help the mind regain its flow.
It **blocks acetylcholinesterase**,
And **butyrylcholinesterase**—a rare two-phase.
So **ACh** can hang around,
To strengthen signals, thought, and sound.
Used for **Alzheimer's disease**,
And **Parkinson's dementia**, where minds freeze.
It gently helps delay the slide,
While keeping function more aligned.
Comes in patch or **oral form**,
The **patch is smooth**, the **GI's warm**.
Nausea, vomiting, are quite a feat,
So start with food if taken to eat.
Side effects? A cholinergic ride:
Bradycardia, fainting, tremors wide.
Weight loss, diarrhea, muscle twitch,
And rarely, **GI bleed** may pitch.
Monitor for cardiac strain,
BP, HR, and weight loss gain.
If GI side effects arrive,
Switch to **patch** to help survive.
Teach patients how to dose with care:
Oral twice daily, meals to share.
The **patch is daily**, upper arm or back,
And **rotate sites** to stay on track.

No black box warning, still observe—
In elders, **falls** may curve the nerve.
And **skin reactions** from the patch
Need checking if they ever catch.
Drug interactions? Few at best—
But don't combine with meds that test
The **cholinergic nervous tide**—
Like **succinylcholine**, side by side.
So **Exelon**, with dual-block might,
Helps keep the brain a bit more bright.
In dementia's fog, it lights a flame,
To hold the line in memory's name.

Part VI
Sleep, Sedatives & Restless Legs

BUTALBITAL/ ACETAMINOPHEN/ CAFFEINE (FIORICET)

Barbiturate Combo - Analgesic / Sedative / Stimulant

When **tension headaches** start to roar,
And simple meds don't help restore,
Fioricet blends a triple crew—
To soothe, sedate, and pull you through.
Butalbital brings a **calming wave**,
A **barbiturate** that helps you brave
The **muscle tension**, stress, and tight—
But it comes with caution, day and night.

Acetaminophen—your pain reliever,
Blocks prostaglandins like a fever weaver.
It eases **aches** from deep inside,
But watch the **liver**—don't let it slide.
Caffeine perks the vessels wide,
Then **clamps them down**, so pain can subside.
It boosts absorption, adds some flair,
And fights the **drowsiness** that Butalbital bears.

It's used for **tension-type headaches** most,
And off-label where **migraine** symptoms host.
But not for **daily use or long**,
Or **rebound headaches** may come on strong.
Side effects can still appear:
**Drowsiness, dizziness, ringing ear,
Nausea, anxiety,** or **GI pain,
Dependence** risk is not so plain.

Monitor for mood and signs
Of **overuse**, which often aligns
With taking too much day by day—
And let the **liver labs** lead the way.
Teach patients: **limit dose per week**,
To **twice or less**, so pain won't peak.
Warn of **withdrawal** if they quit,
And **no alcohol**—not one sip.

No **black box warning**, but take note:
Acetaminophen's liver vote.
Don't mix with more APAP meds,
Or risk **toxicity** in the liver beds.
Drug interactions? Quite a few:
With **sedatives**, it may overdo.
Avoid with **benzos, opioids,** or drink,
And check CYP enzymes when you think.

So **Fioricet**, a combo brew,
Can help—but only if managed true.
It's powerful, yes, but best with grace,
To keep the head in a better place.

ESZOPICLONE (LUNESTA)
Hypnotic / Non-Benzodiazepine Sleep Aid

When **racing thoughts** won't let you rest,
And **counting sheep** won't pass the test,
Eszopiclone comes soft and light,
To **gently guide you into night**.
It's a **non-benzo**, hypnotic class,
But works on **GABA** all the same, with class.
It binds the **BZ1 receptor zone**,
To help the brain shut down and tone.
Used for **insomnia**, short or long,
It helps you **fall asleep and sleep strong**.
Not for naps or restless days—
It's a **nighttime med**, in quiet haze.
Side effects? Let's take a glance:
Bitter taste, dry mouth, sleep trance.
Headache, dizziness, next-day fog,
And rare reports of **sleepwalk jogs**.
More rarely still, **complex sleep acts**—
Like **eating, driving, calling exes back**.
Patients may not recall a thing,
So safety warnings are everything.
Monitor for abuse or change—
Some **dependence** risk is in its range.
And **withdrawal** may bring restless nights,
So **taper slow** if sleep reignites.
Teach patients: take it **right at bed**,
Don't mix with wine or meds that spread
CNS sedation deep—
Or they may fall into unsafe sleep.
Black box warning? Yes, indeed:
For **complex behaviors**—take heed.
Driving, eating, even sex
While fast asleep? What happens next?
Drug interactions? A few worth note:
With **CNS depressants**, change your quote.
Azole antifungals can raise the game,
And **CYP3A4 inhibitors** do the same.
So **Lunesta**, with stardust tone,
Helps minds unwind and rest alone.
But used with care and close insight,
It makes the world feel safe at night.

LORAZEPAM (ATIVAN)

Benzodiazepine / Anxiolytic / Anticonvulsant / Sedative

When **panic climbs** and thoughts won't slow,
And **tension rises** head to toe,
Lorazepam brings soft release—
A **benzo wave** of calming peace.
It **boosts GABA** in the brain's wide sea,
To **depress the CNS** gently.
It calms the mind, slows down the spin,
And helps the stillness grow within.
Used for **anxiety, status seizures**,
Pre-op calm, or **ETOH wean-fevers**.
Also helps with **agitation**'s call—
When peace feels miles from the hall.
Side effects? They come on light:
Drowsiness, dizziness, slowed-down might.
Confusion, weakness, memory blur,
And **falls in elders** may occur.
More serious? **Respiratory fail**,
Especially when **opioids sail**.
Dependency may form in time—
So **short-term use** is more in line.
Black box warning? Yes—it's there:
For use with **opioids**, beware.
Coma, breath suppression, death may rise—
So monitor with cautious eyes.
Monitor sedation, breathing deep,
And **fall risk** if they're on the steep.
Watch for **withdrawal**, if they stop—
As seizures or rebound can suddenly pop.

Teach patients: don't stop on a whim,
Taper slowly from the brim.
Avoid **alcohol** and late-night drive,
Until they know how they'll arrive.
Drug interactions? Quite a few—
With **CNS depressants**, it pulls through.
And watch with drugs that share the lane
Of **liver CYP enzymes** in the brain.
So **Ativan**, though fast and real,
Can calm the mind and help it heal.
But only used with thought and care—
Or risk and peace may both be there.

MIDAZOLAM (NAYZILAM)

Benzodiazepine / Anticonvulsant / Sedative / Nasal Rescue Med

When **seizures strike** without a break,
And silence is too long to make,
Midazolam steps in with speed—
To give the brain the calm it needs.
A **benzodiazepine**, fast and clear,
It calms the nerves and **quiets fear**.
It **boosts GABA**, slows the storm,
And helps the brain return to norm.
Nayzilam is the **nasal spray**,
For **acute seizure clusters** in the fray.
No IV lines or pills to take—
Just spray it once for rescue's sake.
Used in ages 12 and up,
When **intermittent seizures** overflow the cup.
It's **pre-measured, portable**, ready to go—
To stop the surge before it grows.
Side effects? Sedation's first:
Drowsiness, fatigue, or **speech reversed**.
Nasal discomfort, throat may sting,
And **respiratory depression** is a thing.
Monitor breathing after dose,
Especially if another's close.
And know that with **opioids near**,
The risk for **coma** may appear.
Black box warning? Yes, take heed—
For **respiratory risks** in combo need.
With **CNS depressants**, stay alert—
Because this drug can deeply hurt.
Teach caregivers how to give,
And when to call for help to live.
If seizures don't stop after spray one,
A second dose might soon be done.
Drug interactions? Yep, a bunch—
With **alcohol, benzos**, and sedative punch.
Also **CYP3A4** has a hand—
So check what meds they have on hand.
So **Midazolam**, with lightning grace,
Can calm the fire in seizure space.
A rescue med for clusters wild,
That brings relief to brain and child.

TEMAZEPAM (RESTORIL)
Benzodiazepine – Short-Term Sleep Aid

When sleep won't come and nights feel long, And every sound or thought feels wrong, **Temazepam**, a benzo true, Can help the body rest on cue.

It's used for **short-term insomnia**, To hush the noise, remove the drama. It binds to **GABA-A** receptors tight, Enhancing rest throughout the night.

Classified a **Schedule IV**, It's meant for use a few weeks—no more. Dependency can build with time, So caution lies in every line.

Onset hits in about an hour, So take it when you're in sleep's power. Avoid with food, or meals too near, As **delayed effect** can then appear.

Half-life is moderate—longer than some, About **8 to 20 hours** in sum. So grogginess may linger slow, Especially in the **elderly** flow.

Side effects include **confusion**, **Drowsiness**, or **next-day intrusion**. **Memory loss**, and sometimes more— **Sleepwalking**, even out the door.

Don't mix with **alcohol** or meds That also tuck folks into beds. Respiratory depression risk May rise with combos on that list.

Rebound insomnia may come back If stopped abruptly, that's a fact. So always **taper**, never drop, Or withdrawal could make sleep stop.

It's not for patients who might bear A **history of substance care**. Addiction, misuse, and regret— Make sure informed consent is met.

Avoid it in **pregnancy** And those with **COPD**. It may depress the breath at night, And leave you gasping in the light.

Though older, it's still sometimes used, When newer options are refused. But newer meds are often sought, With fewer risks and clearer thought.

Still, when prescribed and used with care, **Temazepam** can help repair The space where rest was lost before— Just use it wisely, nothing more.

SUVOREXANT (BELSOMRA)
Orexin Receptor Antagonist - Insomnia Treatment

When thoughts keep racing through your head, And rest won't come when you're in bed, **Suvorexant** may block the tide, And help the body slip inside.
It works in quite a different way, From **benzos** or the **Z-drug** fray. It blocks **orexin**, not GABA flow— A newer path to make sleep grow.
Orexin keeps us bright and wired, But in insomnia, it's not desired. So Belsomra comes to hush the brain, And ease the **wake-promoting chain**.
It's used for **sleep onset** and **delay**, And keeping sleep from drifting away. But unlike others, with less "kick," Its effects can be a bit more slick.
Take it within **30 before bed**, But only when you're restfully led. Don't eat too close—meals interfere, And **delayed onset** may appear.
Daytime drowsiness can stay, So **fall precautions** lead the way. **Sleep paralysis** may occur, And **vivid dreams** may slightly blur.
Rare but real, some people find **Hallucinations** of eerie kind. Though gentle, still, it must be screened, Especially if **mental health** is gleaned.
CYP3A4 interactions reign— So **azole drugs** may clog the lane. Avoid with **alcohol**, and don't combine With other meds that cross the line.

It's **Schedule IV**, but not as strict, As benzos that the brain can't quit. Still, dependence may arise, So watch for use that multiplies.
Not for **narcolepsy**, that's clear, Since orexin loss is already near. And pregnancy? Not yet advised— More study's needed to be wise.
So if you're tossing every night, And softer meds don't hold you tight, **Suvorexant** may do the trick— By dimming down the **orexin flick**.

SOLRIAMFETOL (SUNOSI)
Wakefulness-Promoting Agent - Narcolepsy & Sleep Apnea Fatigue

When waking up feels like a chore, And naps are needed more and more, **Solriamfetol** brings the spark— To light the mind and lift the dark.

It's not a **stimulant** in the norm, But still it keeps the brain in form. A **dopamine-norepinephrine reuptake block**, To help the **sleep-deprived** restock.

It treats **narcolepsy's deep fatigue**, And **sleep apnea** that cuts intrigue. When CPAP helps but you're still tired, **Sunosi's** path may be inspired.

Its onset hits within an hour, And holds you through the waking power. **Once a day**, by morning light, To boost your mood and mental might.

Side effects you may observe: **Anxiety, nausea, heart rate swerve. Headache, insomnia**, and **dry mouth**, Or **high blood pressure** creeping south.

Avoid in those with **cardiac strain**, Uncontrolled **hypertension pain**. It's not approved for kids or teens, And **MAOI use** is off the scene.

C-IV it's not—surprise, it's free From scheduled class officially. But **abuse potential** is still checked, So prescribers ought to still reflect.

Renal dosing must be tight, Adjust the dose if kidneys fight. Not for folks with **end-stage fail**, So labs will help you set the sail.

No abrupt stop—the fatigue may flare, The body needs a tapered care. But when the weariness runs deep, **Solriamfetol** wakes from sleep.

So if you're dragging through the haze, And can't reclaim your brighter days, Let **Sunosi** help you rise— And greet the sun with open eyes.

HYDROXYZINE (VISTARIL)
Antihistamine - Sleep, Anxiety, and Allergies

An old-school med with many roles, **Hydroxyzine** soothes restless souls. An **antihistamine**, first-gen strong, It helps when sleep or nerves go wrong.
It blocks **H1 receptors** tight, To stop the itch or calm the fright. But more than allergies it tames— It quiets **anxiety's racing flames**.
Vistaril is the name you'll see When used for sleep or therapy. While **Atarax** is often found In allergy bins the world around.
Though not a **benzo**, it still brings rest, A **non-habit forming** calming guest. For **insomnia**, it's often tried When safer routes are bona fide.
It also **reduces pre-op fear**, And calms the mind when danger's near. In panic, grief, or mental strain, It helps reset the anxious brain.
Side effects? They do appear— **Sedation**, **dry mouth**, feeling queer. **Dizziness**, **blurred vision** too, And sometimes a strange mental view.
It starts to work in under one, And lasts for **four to six hours** run. But some report that grog may stay And linger on the following day.
It's **not controlled**, and not abused, So doctors like it safely used. But don't mix with **alcohol** or meds That slow your breath or cloud your heads.
Avoid in those who **prolong QT**, Or with **elder fall risk** history. For pregnant folks, it's Category C, So only used if truly key.
Used **PO**, **IM**, or **capsule deep**, But mostly oral when for sleep. A **25 to 50 mg** dose Is usually where most come close.
So if you're seeking gentle peace, And want the spinning thoughts to cease, Try **Hydroxyzine**—a simple friend, To help the mind and body mend.

ZOLPIDEM (AMBIEN)
Sedative-Hypnotic / GABA-A Agonist / Insomnia Agent

When **sleep won't come** and thoughts won't slow,
And hours drag with nowhere to go,
Zolpidem drifts in like mist—
A whisper on the **GABA list**.
It binds to **GABA-A**, alpha-1,
To help the busy brain feel done.
Not quite a benzo, though close in class,
It calms the waves and lets dreams pass.
Used for **short-term insomnia's spell**,
When nights feel long and not so well.
Ambien tabs or **CR release**,
Or **sublingual** for faster peace.
Side effects? A sleepy tune:
Dizziness, next-day fog, too soon.
Sleepwalking, eating, even **driving**,
Strange behaviors—still surviving.
Black box warning? Yes, it's real:
Complex sleep behaviors that can steal
Safety in the midnight scene—
So take with care, keep routines clean.
Teach patients: take it **right before bed**,
And only when your **head meets head**.
On **empty stomach**, let it flow—
Or it may work **too fast** or **too slow**.
Don't crush CR, and don't repeat
If you wake at 2 and can't re-sleep.
Only take when **7 hours** await,
Or grogginess may be your fate.
Monitor for mood and mind,
And signs of **dependence** you might find.
Rebound insomnia can return
If stopped too fast—let dosing learn.
Drug interactions? CNS crowd—
Benzos, alcohol, all allowed
To stack the sedative effect—
So use with caution and respect.
So **Ambien**, smooth and sleep-designed,
Can quiet the overactive mind.
But always with a cautious plan—
For dreams should **heal**, not **get out of hand**.

Part VII
ADHD, Stimulants & Wakefulness

ARMODAFINIL (NUVIGIL)
Wakefulness-Promoting Agent / CNS Stimulant-Like

When **sleep attacks** at the worst of times,
Armodafinil steps in with chimes.
It boosts **wakefulness**, sharp and clean,
For those who feel they're stuck in dream.
It's used in **narcolepsy, sleep apnea**, too,
And for **shift work sleepiness** that's hard to undo.
Not quite a **stimulant**, but works on the brain,
In ways we don't fully explain
Though **mechanism's** a little obscure,
It **influences dopamine**, that's for sure.
It blocks the **reuptake**, keeps it high,
So you stay alert when hours fly by.
But watch for **side effects** on the list:
Headache, anxiety, can't be missed.
Nausea, dry mouth, maybe **insomnia**,
And **dizziness** that disrupts the panorama
There's a risk for **serious rash**, be warned—
Stevens-Johnson has been mourned.
And rare **angioedema** may appear,
So stop the drug if signs draw near.
Monitor mental health with care—
Watch for **mania, agitation,** or despair.

Assess for **abuse** or **dependency**,
Especially with stimulant tendency.
Tell patients to **avoid late doses**—
Or **sleep will vanish** in high doses.
Warn them about driving, too,
Until they know what the drug will do.
Black box warning? There is none,
But still, respect how fast it runs.
It may **interact** with birth control pills,
Reducing their protective thrills.
Also caution with **CYP3A4**,
Drugs like **ketoconazole**—there's more.
It's **CYP inducers** or inhibitors, too,
That change how **Nuvigil** flows through you.
So **Armodafinil**, sleek and bright,
Brings heavy eyelids back to light.
But handle with a thoughtful plan,
And teach the risks—because you can.

ATOMOXETINE (STRATTERA)
Selective Norepinephrine Reuptake Inhibitor (NRI)

For minds that race or quickly stray,
Atomoxetine clears the way.
It's not a stimulant, yet still bold—
It helps **ADHD** take hold.
It **blocks norepinephrine's reuptake**, neat,
So focus lasts and thoughts repeat.
No dopamine surge, no quick high,
Just calm that helps the day go by.
Approved for **children and adults alike**,
When **stimulants** cause too much spike.
It builds up slow—so give it time,
Effects may show by week two's climb.
Side effects? Yes, some to know:
Dry mouth, **GI upset**, **mood swings** grow.
Insomnia, **fatigue**, **urinary hold**,
And in some teens, emotions cold
Watch for **suicidal thought or cry**,
Especially when starting—stay close by.
Also risk of **liver injury**, rare—
Check **jaundice**, **dark urine**, and beware.
Monitor heart rate and BP trend,
As **hypertension** can ascend.
Track **mood**, **sleep**, and appetite drop,
And know when med adjustments pop.
Teach patients it won't work right away,
But give it time—it builds each day.
Avoid abrupt stop—**taper slow**,
And take it **daily**, high or low.
Black box warning does apply:
For **suicidal risk in youth**, keep eye.
Especially in **first few weeks**,
Supportive care is what one seeks.
Drug **interactions**? Yes indeed—
With **MAOIs**, halt—dangerous speed.
Caution with **albuterol**, **pressors**, too,
And **CYP2D6 inhibitors** alter what it'll do.
So **Strattera** finds its mindful place,
With slower steps and steady pace.
A thoughtful med, when used with care,
To bring attention back to air.

DEXEDRINE (DEXTROAMPHETAMINE SULFATE)

CNS Stimulant - ADHD & Narcolepsy

Dexedrine is its classic name, An **amphetamine** that fuels the brain. A legacy med, still used today, For **ADHD** and sleep delay.
It boosts both **dopamine** and **norepinephrine**, To sharpen focus, hold attention in. In **narcolepsy**, it brings back spark, And pushes through the mental dark.
It's **Schedule II**, so tightly bound, With **abuse potential** that's well renowned. It gives the mind a sharper edge, But only near the therapeutic ledge.
It comes in **tablet, spanule**, too, The latter's extended to get you through. **Immediate release** acts real fast, But **extended** versions longer last.
In **ADHD**, it helps the mind To organize and stay aligned. For **school-age kids** or working peers, It's helped for decades through the years.
Side effects you should know and teach: **Appetite loss**, **dry mouth**, speech. **Insomnia**, **irritability**, And **tachycardia**, potentially.
Growth suppression may occur— So **track height and weight** to infer. Take **early in the day**, not late, Or sleep may suffer from its state. Avoid with meds that raise the strain, Like **MAOIs**—that brings great pain. And those with **heart conditions**, too, May find the risks outweigh the view.

Monitor for **misuse signs**: Taking more than given lines. Crushing, snorting, skipping school— Means it's time to change the rule.
It's metabolized in **the liver**, So screen for meds that make it quiver. And those with **substance use** before Should tread with care and close the door.
Though newer brands are on the rise, Like **Adderall** in different guise, **Dexedrine** still plays its part— A stimulant with an older heart.

SOLRIAMFETOL (SUNOSI)
Wakefulness-Promoting Agent - Narcolepsy & Sleep Apnea Fatigue

When heavy eyes just won't obey, And sleep attacks steal half your day, **Solriamfetol**, known as **Sunosi**, Can help you feel a little more rosy. It treats the fog that will not lift, When **narcolepsy** starts to drift. And if with CPAP you still yawn, This med can help you power on.

It's not a classic stimulant, But still enhances brain ascent. It blocks **dopamine** and **NE reuptake**, To sharpen thought and keep you awake.

Approved for use in adults who feel **Sleep apnea**'s fatigue is real— Even when treated, if tiredness lingers, **Sunosi** steps in with gentle fingers. It starts to work in **one quick hour**, Its **half-life** gives a lasting power. One dose **each morning**, early planned, To keep you focused, sharp, and spanned.

Side effects you might observe: **Anxiety**, **headache**, energy swerve. **Nausea**, **dry mouth**, **BP rise**, And **insomnia** in some replies.

It's **not a controlled substance** yet, But misuse risk is still a threat. So watch for those who chase the boost— And keep your oversight well-loosed.

Avoid with other **dopamine drugs**, Like **MAOIs** or risky plugs. And always check the **renal base**— Dose adjust for kidney space.

Don't give to folks with **high blood pressure**, Uncontrolled risk makes outcomes lesser. Monitor **heart rate**, **vitals**, too— This med is strong and must stay true.

Withdrawal symptoms can appear If stopped too fast — so taper clear. And don't take late within the day, Or sleep might wander far away. Still, when **narcolepsy** takes hold, Or tired days feel gray and cold, **Solriamfetol** can break the chain— And help you live with clearer brain.

DEXMETHYLPHENIDATE (FOCALIN)
CNS Stimulant / ADHD Agent

When focus fades and minds won't stay,
Dexmethylphenidate clears the way.
It's the **d-threo form**—the active slice,
Of **methylphenidate**—extra precise.
A **CNS stimulant**, sleek and fast,
It helps **ADHD** thoughts hold fast.
By blocking **dopamine, norepinephrine**'s reuptake,
It sharpens brains that feel half-awake.
It's used for **attention** that slips and sways,
In **kids and adults** through hectic days.
It boosts the brain's executive tune,
From dawn until the afternoon.
Side effects can pack a punch:
Insomnia, anxiety, skipping lunch.
Weight loss, dry mouth, racing heart,
And **tics** or **nervousness** may start.
More rare but serious signs include:
Psychosis, mania, altered mood.
Hypertension, or **cardiac strain**,
So screen for issues in heart or brain.
Monitor height and weight in youth,
And track **BP, HR**, and sleep truth.
Check for signs of **abuse** or **craving**,
And any mood that feels worth saving.

Teach patients: **take in the AM**, not late,
Or sleep may never find the gate.
Don't **crush the XR**—swallow whole,
And don't play games with dosage control.
Black box warning? Yes—be aware:
Of **abuse potential** hiding there.
It's a **Schedule II**, so monitor tight,
And use only as prescribed, day or night.
Drug interactions? Yes, take heed:
With **MAOIs**, it's a dangerous speed.
Also beware **acidic foods**—
They lower how the med gets used.
So **Focalin**, sharp and focused fire,
Can help the restless brain aspire.
With careful hands and guided flow,
It helps attention bloom and grow.

DEXTROAMPHETAMINE/ AMPHETAMINE (ADDERALL)

CNS Stimulant / ADHD & Narcolepsy Agent

When **focus drifts** and thoughts collide,
And energy's hard to summon inside,
Adderall steps in—strong and bright,
To turn the mental fog to light.
It's a mix of **dextro** and **levo** base,
Amphetamine salts—a classic case.
They boost **dopamine** and **norepinephrine**,
To get the brain back in the spin
Used for **ADHD** in kids and grown,
And **narcolepsy**, when sleep is overblown.
It sharpens tasks and keeps things clear,
With mental gears that grind to gear.
Side effects may show up fast:
Insomnia, **loss of weight**, won't last.
Tachycardia, **BP rise**,
And **jitters dancing in the eyes**.
Also risk of **mood decline**,
With **anxiety**, or even **rage in line**.
Long-term use can wear things thin—
With **tolerance**, or **crashes** that begin.
Monitor weight and growth in youth,
Watch for **sleep** and emotional truth.
Check for **cardiac conditions** past,
Before this med is given fast.

Teach patients to take it **early in day**,
And **never double** a dose that may stray.
No crushing XR, and avoid the brew—
Caffeine or alcohol won't play nice too.
Black box warning stands up tall:
For **abuse, addiction**, and sudden fall.
In **those with heart defects**, beware—
There's **risk of death** with stimulant care.
Drug interactions? A decent list:
MAOIs, a fatal twist.
Also caution with **acidic food**,
Which alters how it's understood.
So **Adderall**, a sharp-edged tool,
Helps wandering minds to follow rule.
But wield it with respect and plan,
To serve the brain—not let it span.

GUANFACINE (INTUNIV)
Alpha-2A Adrenergic Agonist / ADHD & Antihypertensive Agent

When **impulses race** and focus slides,
And **restless minds** can't take the rides,
Guanfacine helps the thoughts align,
By slowing down that **mental climb**.
It's an **alpha-2A agonist**,
That calms the brain and clenches fist.
It **reduces sympathetic tone**,
So kids and teens feel more at home.

Used for **ADHD**, not the kind
That craves a stimulant-sharpened mind.
It's for the kids who need the slow—
Hyperactive, impulsive flow.
Also used for **blood pressure drops**,
Though less now since newer swaps.
And in **Tourette's** or **autistic strain**,
It may reduce the **rage or pain**.

Side effects? A sleepy slide:
Sedation, drowsy, low HR ride.
Hypotension, dizziness, too,
And **dry mouth** may come into view.
More rare, but worth the look:
Bradycardia may write the book.
And if stopped **suddenly**, take care—
Rebound hypertension could be there.

Monitor for blood pressure dips,
And **heart rate changes** in your scripts.
Start it **low and slow**, then rise,
To help avoid those sleepy sighs.
Teach patients: take it **once a day**,
At bedtime if they feel the sway.
Don't crush XR, swallow whole,
And taper off to meet the goal.

No black box warning, though it's smart
To watch for **mood shifts** or slow start.
It may **enhance sedation** paired
With **CNS depressants** shared.
Drug interactions? Some to note:
With **valproate**, it gets a vote.
Can raise **guanfacine levels high**,
So monitor if mood swings fly.

So **Intuniv**, soft and calm and clear,
Brings quiet to the mental sphere.
It smooths the spikes and tones the day,
In a gentle, non-stimulating way.

LISDEXAMFETAMINE (VYVANSE)

CNS Stimulant / ADHD & Binge Eating Disorder Agent

When **focus slips** and **thoughts run wild**,
And every task feels like a trial,
Lisdexamfetamine brings control—
To help the mind regain its role.
It's a **prodrug** form, so nice and neat,
Of **dextroamphetamine**, once complete.
Converted slowly, smooth and clean,
To give a **steady stimulant scene**.
Used for **ADHD**, both young and grown,
To help them **focus**, stay in zone.
Also treats **binge eating** stride,
When urges swell and hide inside.
Side effects? A common stack:
Decreased appetite, sleep thrown back.
Dry mouth, headache, irritation, Tachycardia, and **constipation**.
Anxiety, sweating, or **jittery nerves**,
And in some, **emotional swerves**.
Rarely: **psychosis, mania**, too—
So watch for changes breaking through.
Monitor: heart rate, BP climb,
Growth in children over time.
And screen for **misuse, diversion**, risk—
It's **Schedule II**, not on a whim list.
Teach patients: take it **early in day**,
So **insomnia** won't come to play.
Don't crush or chew—just swallow whole,
And **store it safely**, that's the goal.
Black box warning? Yes, it's true:
For **abuse, dependence**, coming through.
Long-term use without good check
Can put the heart and mind at wreck.
Drug interactions? Watch the stack—
MAOIs must step far back.
And with **acidic food or juice**,
Absorption may turn slightly loose.
So **Vyvanse**, steady, long, and clear,
Helps bring the wandering mind near.
A focused tool when used with care,
To help attention stay right there.

METHYLPHENIDATE (RITALIN, CONCERTA)
CNS Stimulant / ADHD & Narcolepsy Agent

When **focus drifts** and thoughts mislead,
And tasks go missing at lightning speed,
Methylphenidate brings things back—
A **dopamine boost** to stay on track.
It blocks the **reuptake gates** so clean,
For **dopamine** and **norepinephrine's** stream.
The **prefrontal cortex** feels the shift—
With sharpened thoughts and mental lift.
Used in **ADHD**, both young and grown,
And in **narcolepsy**, often shown.
It comes as **IR, ER**, and more—
From **Ritalin** tabs to **Concerta's core**.
Side effects may tag along:
Insomnia, nervousness, heartbeat strong.
Decreased appetite, weight loss, too,
And sometimes mood swings breaking through.
Tics, headaches, and **GI pain**,
Or **BP rising** in the vein.
And though it helps attention's flame,
It sometimes stokes the **anxiety game**.
Monitor growth in kids each year,
And **BP, HR**, keep them near.
Screen for **abuse** and **dependence signs**,
And check for changes in their lines.
Teach patients: take it **early in day**,
So sleep can still come out to play.
Don't crush ER tabs, swallow whole,
And keep the dosing in control.
Black box warning? Yes, for real:
Abuse, misuse, and how they feel.
Can lead to **dependency**, or worse,
So use with care and chart each verse.
Drug interactions? Yes, beware:
MAOIs—don't go there.
Caution with **antihypertensives** too,
It might reduce what they can do.
So **Methylphenidate**, quick and bright,
Can help the **ADHD** take flight.
But only when it's used with care,
To lift the mind and keep it fair.

MODAFINIL (PROVIGIL)

Wakefulness-Promoting Agent / CNS Stimulant-Like / Narcolepsy & Sleep Disorder Therapy

When **daytime sleep** won't let you be,
And rest invades productivity,
Modafinil lights up the way,
To help you **wake and face the day**.
It's not quite like your classic speed—
No **amphetamine** or **dopamine greed**.
It **activates the brain's alerting net**,
Though how it works? Not fully set.
Used for **narcolepsy**, plain and true,
And **sleep apnea** when the mask is through.
Also helps in **shift work strain**,
When circadian clocks misfire the brain.
Side effects? They're mostly tame:
Headache, nausea, and **insomnia's flame**.
Anxiety, dry mouth, dizzy spell,
And sometimes **rash** that doesn't dwell.
But hold up—rare reactions may arise,
Like **Stevens-Johnson**—a big surprise.
So teach patients: if **rash appears**,
Stop the med and shift the gears.
Monitor for mood swings, quick—
It may bring **mania** to the mix.
Check for **BP** and mental tone,
And see how sleep patterns have grown.

Teach patients: take it **in the morn**,
So **sleep at night** won't feel forlorn.
And if it's for **shift work sleep**,
Take it **an hour before** that leap.
No black box warning, but be wise,
Watch for **overuse** in bright disguise.
It's **Schedule IV**, with some abuse,
Though far less than its stimulant use.
Drug interactions? A modest few:
It's a **CYP3A4 inducer**, too.
So **oral contraceptives** may fail—
Back up birth control without fail.
So **Modafinil**, cool and bright,
Helps chase away the sleepy night.
With measured use and rhythm strong,
It helps the weary brain hold on.

Part VIII
Depression, Anxiety & Mood Stabilizers

AMITRIPTYLINE (ELAVIL)
Tricyclic Antidepressant (TCA)

An old-school drug with many roles,
Amitriptyline soothes hurting souls.
A **TCA**, it blocks reuptake tight—
Of **norepinephrine** and **serotonin's light**.
It helps with **depression**, dark and deep,
And **nerve pain** that disturbs your sleep.
For **migraines**, **fibro**, or even **grief**,
This med can sometimes bring relief.

But side effects? Oh yes, a list:
Dry mouth, blurred sight, a **constipated twist**.
Weight gain, fatigue, and **drowsy heads**,
And weird **dreams** while tucked in beds.
Orthostatic drops, and fast heart rates,
Urinary retention complicates.
And don't forget the **QT stretch**,
That heart arrhythmias may catch.

Monitor ECGs with care,
Especially if risk is there.
Liver function, mental state,
And **suicidal thoughts**—don't wait.
Teach patients: **take it at night**,
It may bring on some morning light.
Avoid with **alcohol**, or any brew,
And **sun protection**—yes, that too.

Black box warning stands in view:
For **suicidal thoughts** in youth—stay true.
Especially those **under 25**,
Keep them close, and keep alive.
Interactions? Many, friend:
MAOIs—that's a dangerous blend.
SSRIs may cause **serotonin storm**,
And **CNS depressants** are far from norm.

So **Amitriptyline**, kind but sly,
Can help the pain or make you cry.
Used with care and patient grace,
It finds its proper, healing place.

ARMODAFINIL (NUVIGIL)
Wakefulness-Promoting Agent - Narcolepsy, Sleep Apnea, Shift Work Disorder

When drowsy days just won't let go, And nights at work feel painfully slow, **Armodafinil** brings the lift— A focused, gentle, stimulant shift.

It treats **narcolepsy's deep fatigue**, And **sleep apnea** that drains intrigue. Also helps with **shift work nights**, When circadian rhythm picks its fights.

It's the **R-enantiomer**, pure and clean, Of **modafinil**, its older twin. It lasts a bit longer through the day, With fewer peaks and smoother sway.

The **mechanism** is not well known, But it affects the brain's **dopamine tone**. It blocks reuptake at the gate, To keep you sharp, alert, and straight.

It's **Schedule IV**, so mild but tracked, Less risky than the old amp act. Still, misuse could take its toll, So use with care and clear control.

Once a day, and early on— If taken late, your sleep is gone. Use for **narcolepsy**, **OSA**, Or **shift work disorder** night or day.

Side effects you might expect: **Headache**, **dry mouth**, or **sleep defect**. **Nausea**, **anxiety**, sometimes **rash**, Though most resolve without a clash.

Rarely, it may cause a scare— A **severe rash** or **angioedema** flare. So discontinue at first red sign, And seek a different wake-up line.

Interactions do exist, With **CYP enzymes** on the list. It may affect **birth control pills**, So use a backup to prevent spills.

Avoid in patients with heart strain, Like **LVH** or **valvular pain**. And always monitor mood shifts strong, In case of **mania** come along.

It's not meant for curing sleep, Just helps you **function**, drive, and keep. The cause of tiredness must be known— Before **Nuvigil** is ever shown.

So if your eyelids fight the sun, And work or illness steals the run, Then **Armodafinil** may rise— To bring you back with open eyes.

BUSPIRONE (BUSPAR)
Anxiolytic - Non-Benzo Anxiety Relief

When worry climbs and won't let go, But **benzos** feel a risky show, There's **Buspirone**, a gentler guide— To ease the anxious waves inside.

It's **not a sedative** in the norm, No heavy fog, no tranquil form. It binds **5-HT1A receptors** tight, To dial down stress and calm the fight.

Used for **generalized anxiety**, Without the **CNS toxicity**. No euphoria, no abuse— A cleaner tool for daily use.

Its effects are slow, so don't expect That instant calm some folks detect. It takes about **two to four weeks**, Before the steady stillness peaks.

Dizziness, nausea, dry mouth, light— Those are side effects in sight. But it won't sedate or knock you down, And doesn't make you sleep or frown.

No **withdrawal risk**, no craving ache, So **long-term use** is safer to take. It's not controlled, no DEA class— Just caution when the kidneys pass.

Take it **twice or three times daily**, With or without meals, just plainly. But take it **same time every day**, So blood levels don't drift away.

It does **not interact** with booze, But don't assume it's safe to use. And with **MAOIs**, there's a block— Hypertension risk may shock.

It's not for panic or fast fear, Where **benzos** or **beta-blockers** steer. But for **steady tension**, long and drawn, **Buspirone** is calmly strong.

If switching off a benzo grip, **Overlap** for a safer trip. Then taper down the sedative— Let **Buspar** take the reins and live.

So when anxiety's always near, But **controlled meds** feel unclear, This gentle route may help reset— With **Buspirone**, no major threat.

SELEGILINE (ELDEPRYL, ZELAPAR)

MAO-B Inhibitor – Parkinson's Disease & Depression Adjunct

When dopamine begins to fall, And tremors answer every call, **Selegiline** steps in to fight, To keep the motor system right.
It's a **monoamine oxidase B** block, To stop **dopamine's** ticking clock. By slowing how it's torn away, It helps the brain prolong the day.
Used in early **Parkinson's care**, To hold off levodopa's wear. Or as an add-on down the line, To boost the meds and hold the spine.
Also used in **depression**, rare— But only when folks do not fare On SSRIs or newer meds, **MAOIs** step in instead.
The form depends on patient flow: **Eldepryl** is the **oral go**, While **Zelapar** dissolves and stays **Sublingual** in its rapid phase.
Watch for **insomnia**—very clear— It's **stimulating**, not too near To bedtime, or the night's undone— Take it **early with the sun**.
Side effects? They may include: **Nausea, dizzy**, altered mood. And though it's B-selective now, At higher doses, breaks that vow.
At high enough, it blocks **MAO-A**, And that's when **cheese effects** may play. So tyramine can then provoke **Hypertensive crises** stroke.
Avoid with **SSRIs, SNRI meds**, And **tramadol**, or **serotonin heads**. The **washout period** must be planned, Or **serotonin syndrome** gets out of hand.
May **increase dyskinesia** too, When paired with **levodopa's crew**. So watch the movement, gait, and tone— Adjust if tremors overblown.
In **pregnancy**, the risks aren't clear, So weigh the needs with caution near. And never give with uncontrolled **Thyroid issues** or hearts too bold.
It's not a cure, but slows the pace, Gives Parkinson's a steadier race. And though it's older, still it stands, **Selegiline** lends healing hands.

SELEGILINE PATCH (EMSAM)

MAOI – Depression-Specific, Transdermal Route

When nothing lifts the heavy haze, And **MDD** still clouds your days, The **Selegiline patch**, called **Emsam**, might Help turn the dark to shades of light.

It's a **monoamine oxidase B** block, But at high doses, turns the lock On **MAO-A** as well, to keep More **serotonin**, **NE**, and **dopamine** deep. It boosts the brain's depleted stores, Through **transdermal** means—no guts, no chores. No **first-pass liver**, no GI trip, Just steady flow through skin and strip.

It's applied **once daily**, clean and dry, To hip or upper torso, thigh. Rotate the site and hold it tight, But don't apply where clothes rub tight.

At **6 mg**, there's **no food rule**, But **9 or 12 mg** breaks that school. Then **tyramine-rich foods** must go— Or **hypertensive crises** grow.

No **aged cheese**, no **cured meat bites**, No **red wine**, **soy sauce**, foodie nights. Avoid **fermented** treats and beer, Or blood pressure may spike with fear.

Side effects can still appear: **Insomnia**, **agitation**, fear. **Headache**, **nausea**, weight loss too, And **skin reactions** at the glue. **Serotonin syndrome** is a risk, With **SSRIs** or **tramadol** mixed. So always give a **washout span**, And taper slowly, per the plan.

It's **not for kids** or teens in strife, And **bipolar** may bring manic life. So screen for mood swings in the past, Before prescribing this at last.

In **elder adults**, start low and slow, As blood pressure may drop or grow. And **orthostatic risks** may rise, So watch them carefully with eyes.

It's **not a first-line choice** today, But for **resistant MDD**, it may Be worth the try when hope runs thin— Emsam lets new strength begin.

So if depression won't retreat, And other meds have faced defeat, The **Selegiline patch** might be the key— To bring back light and clarity.

DULOXETINE (CYMBALTA)

SNRI - Serotonin-Norepinephrine Reuptake Inhibitor

When **pain and mood** both weigh the day,
Duloxetine can clear the way.
It blocks reuptake, strong and sure,
Of **serotonin** and **norepinephrine's** cure.
An **SNRI**, it pulls dual weight—
For **depression, anxiety**, and chronic state.
Neuropathic pain, fibro, too,
And **MSK aches** that won't bid adieu
Used for **MDD, GAD**, and more,
And **diabetic nerve pain** at its core.
It lifts the mood and eases sting,
While keeping mental balance in swing.
Side effects? A decent list:
Dry mouth, nausea, sweaty mist.
Drowsiness, fatigue, or just **insomnia**,
Appetite may shift (or drop ya)
Sexual dysfunction may arrive,
And **BP** might begin to drive.
There's also risk of **SI thoughts**,
Especially in younger age slots.
Monitor BP and mood real close,
Especially when starting the dose.
Watch for **serotonin syndrome signs**—
Like **fever, rigid**, or **confused lines**.
Teach patients not to **stop too fast**,
Taper slow so withdrawal won't blast.

They may feel **brain zaps, dizzy, numb**,
So stopping quick is never the sum.
Black box warning—yes, it's bold:
Suicidal thoughts in the young and old.
Particularly in **patients under 25**,
Close support keeps them alive.
Drug interactions? Yes, a few:
MAOIs are a major no-go crew.
Tramadol, St. John's Wort, SSRIs,
May raise serotonin to the skies.
So **Cymbalta**, when used with grace,
Can help both **mind and body** embrace.
For pain and mood, it's double-wise,
With care, support, and watchful eyes.

MILNACIPRAN (SAVELLA)
SNRI - Serotonin-Norepinephrine Reuptake Inhibitor / Fibromyalgia Agent

When **fibro pain** won't fade or break,
And every touch feels like an ache,
Milnacipran helps shift the tide—
To **calm the nerves that scream inside.**
It's not for mood like others seem,
Though **SNRI** is still its theme.
It **blocks reuptake** of **serotonin**,
And **norepinephrine**—steady tonin'.

Used to treat **fibromyalgia's storm**,
To help the brain **reprocess pain's form**.
Not approved for **depression** (unlike kin),
But helps **fatigue** and **ache within**.
Side effects can take their turn:
Nausea, sweating, heartburn burn.
Headache, dizziness, dry mouth, too,
And **increased heart rate** may break through.

Also risk of **mood decline**,
So screen for **suicide signs** in line.
And **BP** may climb or hold on tight—
So monitor it morning and night.
Teach patients: take it twice a day,
And titrate slow to keep side effects at bay.
Don't stop abruptly—taper wise,
To avoid withdrawal's sharp surprise.

Black box warning? Not assigned,
But **suicidal thoughts** still underline.
Especially in **younger minds**,
Keep support close and watch the signs.
Drug interactions? Yes, take note:
With **MAOIs**, don't rock the boat.
And with **serotonergic meds** in play,
Serotonin syndrome may come your way.

So **Savella**, with dual-track grace,
Can help calm pain and slow the race.
It lifts the fog, resets the tone,
And helps those hurting feel less alone.

NORTRIPTYLINE (PAMELOR)

Tricyclic Antidepressant (TCA) / Neuropathic Pain & Depression Agent

When **nerve pain burns** or **moods run low**,
And **sleep feels far**, and thoughts move slow,
Nortriptyline steps in the lane—
To help reset the **aching brain**.
A **TCA**, from older days,
But still it shines in **useful ways**.
It blocks the **reuptake** of **norepinephrine**,
And **serotonin**, to boost what's within.
Used for **depression**, often masked,
But now in **chronic pain** it's tasked.
Like **neuropathy, fibro**, or tension swell—
It helps the nerves play calm and well.
Side effects? Quite a few:
Dry mouth, blurred vision, constipation too.
Urine retention, drowsy fog,
And sometimes that **TCA weight gain slog**.
Orthostatic hypotension might arise,
And in the elders—**fall risk** applies.
Also watch for **mood to dip**,
Especially when starting the script.
Black box warning? Yes—be aware:
Suicidal thoughts may linger there.
Especially in the young or teen,
So monitor closely, keep it seen.
Monitor: EKG before you start,
If patient's got a **cardiac heart**.

Because **QT prolongation** and arrhythmias
Can be part of TCAs' previous.
Teach patients: don't stop too quick,
Or **withdrawal** symptoms can make them sick.
Taper slow, and take with care,
Usually **at bedtime**, if they're aware.
Drug interactions? Yes, indeed—
MAOIs? That's a dangerous speed.
And caution with **CYP2D6** drugs,
It may increase levels or cause some bugs.
So **Pamelor**, though old-school styled,
Still helps the hurting and the riled.
With gentle dose and steady view,
It brings relief to quite a few.

PIMAVANSERIN (NUPLAZID)
Selective Serotonin Inverse Agonist / Parkinson's Disease Psychosis Agent

When **visions rise** and voices call,
And **Parkinson's minds** begin to stall,
Pimavanserin clears the haze—
To help the **psychosis** drift away.
It's not your standard antipsych,
No dopamine block to jam the mic.
It works on **5-HT$_2$A**,
As an **inverse agonist**, leading the way.
It **tones down serotonin's excess**,
In **Parkinson's Disease Psychosis distress**.
Without the risk of worsening gait,
Or freezing steps that meds create.
Used for PD psychosis only,
Where minds grow scared, or nights feel lonely.
Hallucinations, delusions too—
It helps the world feel more like you.
Side effects? A few may show:
QT prolongation, heart rate low.
Peripheral edema, nausea, falls,
And **confusion** in some patient calls.
Monitor EKG before,
Especially if they've heart risk or more.
No dopaminergic impact here—
Which keeps it safe for movement fear.
Teach patients: take it **once a day**,
With or without food, okay.
No titration—start full dose,
And **don't stop fast**, or symptoms coast.

Black box warning? Yes—take heed:
For **increased mortality** risk indeed.
In **elderly dementia psychosis**,
Other causes lead to losses.
Drug interactions? CYP on file—
3A4 inhibitors can compile.
Avoid with strong ones like **ketoconazole**,
Or reduce the dose if they're in the call.
So **Nuplazid**, gentle, clear, and wise,
Brings calm to **Parkinson's haunted skies**.
A niche, refined, and mindful tool,
To bring back peace where fears once rule.

Part IX
Muscle Relaxants, Motion & Myasthenia

BACLOFEN (LIORESAL)
Muscle Relaxant – GABA-B Agonist

When **spastic limbs** are stiff with strain,
Baclofen helps to ease the pain.
It works through **GABA-B**, nice and slow,
To **calm the nerves** and let movement flow.
Used for **spasticity**, from **MS** or **SCI**,
To loosen tight muscles that won't comply.
It quiets signals down the spine,
To help the body re-align.

Side effects? A sleepy list:
Drowsiness, dizziness, nausea's twist.
Weakness, fatigue, and **confused mood**,
Sometimes **low BP**, or **clumsiness** too.
With **long-term use**, withdrawal's real—
Hallucinations, seizures, that's the deal.
Taper slow—don't stop too fast,
Or rebound spasms may come back fast.

Monitor mental status and gait,
Check for **falls** or a **sedated state**.
Also track **renal function**, dear,
Since **clearance drops** when kidneys veer.
Teach patients not to drink or drive,
Until they know how they'll survive.
Avoid abrupt withdrawal, warn—
Especially if intrathecal form is worn.

Black box warning makes it plain:
Stopping intrathecal Baclofen brings pain.
Organ failure, rhabdo, or **death**,
So taper it slow—protect each breath.
Interactions come into play
With **CNS depressants** every day—
Like **benzos, opioids,** even **booze**,
All amplify the sleepy fuse.

So **Baclofen**, a calming friend,
Helps spastic muscles stretch and bend.
But guide its use with care and grace,
To keep the patient in a safer place.

DANTROLENE (DANTRIUM)

Direct-Acting Skeletal Muscle Relaxant / Ryanodine Receptor Antagonist

When **muscles seize** and burn like flame,
Dantrolene steps into the game.
It acts **directly on the cell**,
To cool the storm and break the spell.
It blocks the **ryanodine receptor gate**,
Reducing **calcium's exit rate**.
No calcium? No muscle fire—
It stops the **rigid, seizing wire**.
Used for **malignant hyperthermia**, fast,
And **spasticity** when tension's vast.
Also treats **neuroleptic heat**,
That **NMS**—where muscle and temp compete.
Side effects? Some you'll see:
Drowsiness, dizziness, fatigue, maybe.
Muscle weakness—a trade-off true,
And **diarrhea** may join the crew.
There's also risk with long-term use—
Liver damage may cut loose.
So keep your eye on **LFTs**,
Especially after weeks or threes.
Monitor the patient's tone,
And **temperature** if crisis is known.
Have it ready **peri-op**,
When **succinylcholine** may make heat pop.

Teach patients: watch for **yellow skin**,
Dark urine means it's time to check in.
Don't drive or lift until they see
How much this drug affects their spree.
Black box warning—yes, it's clear:
Hepatotoxicity is the fear.
Especially in **females over 35**,
On long-term use—keep the liver alive.
Drug interactions? A few to name:
With **CNS depressants**, it's much the same.
And watch out if the patient's on
Calcium channel blockers—might prolong.
So **Dantrolene**, a niche but bold,
Can **save a life** when muscles fold.
It cools the fire, slows the shake,
And helps the body **not to break**.

EDROPHONIUM (TENSILON)

Acetylcholinesterase Inhibitor - Myasthenia Gravis Diagnosis

When muscles fade and weakness grows, And no one's sure where function goes, **Edrophonium** takes the lead, To test if **MG** is the need. It blocks the enzyme **AChE**, So more **acetylcholine** can be Released at **neuromuscular sites**, Restoring strength in brief highlights.

It's used in the **Tensilon test**, To see if weakness can be pressed. A sudden lift, though short and fast, Means **myasthenia** may be cast. Given **IV**, a **test dose first**, To catch reactions at their worst. Then a larger one if safe— To check if strength comes back in place.

You'll see **ptosis lift** or grip restore, For seconds, maybe one minute more. If so, the test is called **positive**, Suggesting MG's narrative. But risks are real—this drug is bold, It slows the heart and breaks the mold. **Bradycardia**, **hypotension**, too, **Respiratory arrest** may ensue. That's why you always **give with care**, And keep **atropine** standing there. It's the reversal just in case The heart decides to slow its pace.

It's **not used long-term** anymore, Just diagnosis, nothing more. Newer agents fill the gap For therapy, in modern map.

It may confuse with **cholinergic crises**, Where symptoms mimic MG's slices. So tests must match the full profile— Don't guess just from a single trial.

Contraindications do exist, Like **cardiac disease** on the list. Asthma, ulcers, vagal tone— Could make this test a danger zone.

So now it's rarely used, it's true, But still on exams it waits for you. For classic signs and old-school flair, **Tensilon** has its rightful share. When **MG** is in the air, And eyelids fall with weighted stare, A quick **Edrophonium push** might tell If **acetylcholine** serves them well.

EFGARTIGIMOD (VYVGART)

FcRn Blocker – Myasthenia Gravis Treatment

A brand new way to treat the fight, When **autoantibodies** dim the light. **Efgartigimod**, called **Vyvgart** too, Is changing how we help push through.

It's used for **myasthenia gravis**, Especially those **AChR+** status. When **antibodies** block the nerve, This med helps strength and hope preserve.

It blocks the **neonatal FcRn**, A receptor where IgGs run. By **lowering autoantibody stay**, It clears the path for nerves to play.

Given **IV once per week**, For **four doses**, then we peek. Repeat if symptoms still persist, But only when the docs insist.

It's **not a cure**, but buys some grace, Improves the function, slows the pace. Better grip and breathing seen, In those for whom MG's been mean.

Side effects are mild but real: **Respiratory infections** top the deal. **Headache**, **UTI**, **fatigue** may show, And sometimes **rash** or **GI flow**.

No live vaccines while on the drip, The immune shield has a missing zip. So pause or plan your vaccine course, Before you start this treatment force.

It's not for all—must be **AChR+**, That antibody must show up thus. The test comes first to know the fit, Before the first infusion hit.

It's **well-tolerated**, fairly sleek, And doesn't cause the peaks or leaks Like steroids or immune attacks— Just clears the harmful IgG tracks.

It's not used in **kids** or **pregnancy**, No safety data, yet to see. Still, for adults with MG grind, **Vyvgart** brings a brighter mind.

From **IVIG** to plasmapheresis, Old options often brought new pieces. But now a **targeted approach** is near— With **Efgartigimod**, strength reappears.

MECLIZINE (ANTIVERT)

Antihistamine / Antiemetic / Antivertigo Agent

When **spinning rooms** and **nausea rise**,
And balance leaves your ears and eyes,
Meclizine comes in calm and fast,
To **settle motion** that won't pass.
It's a **first-gen antihistamine**,
With **anticholinergic** routine.
It blocks **H1 receptors** true,
And calms the signals passing through.

Used for **vertigo**, **motion sick**,
And **nausea** that comes on quick.
It's helpful in **inner ear distress**,
Where **vestibular nerves** digress.
Side effects? A sleepy bunch:
Drowsiness, **dry mouth**, slower punch.
Blurred vision, **urine hesitance**,
And sometimes **confusion** at a glance.

In elders, it may cloud the day—
So **fall precautions** lead the way.
And with **BPH** or **glaucoma signs**,
Use caution in those fragile lines.
Monitor sedation and alert,
Especially when driving or at work.
And **teach patients** when to take it best—
One hour before a motion test.

No black box warning, safe in class,
But still go slow, don't dose too fast.
And don't combine with other meds
That make the brain feel filled with lead.
Drug interactions? Yes, a few—
With **alcohol**, it'll double the view.
Other CNS depressants, too,
Can make them stumble more than due.

So **Meclizine**, a travel friend,
Helps nausea, spinning, gently end.
With thoughtful use and patient plan,
It helps restore where balance ran.

TIZANIDINE (ZANAFLEX)

Alpha-2 Adrenergic Agonist / Muscle Relaxant / Spasticity Agent

When **muscles spasm**, tight and sore,
And **neuro pain** makes movements war,
Tizanidine brings gentle grace—
To help those **twitching nerves** embrace.
It's an **alpha-2 agonist**, calm and smooth,
That tells the **spinal cord** to soothe.
It reduces **tone and reflex fire**,
And helps release the tightness wire.
Used for **spasticity** caused by strain,
From **MS, stroke**, or **spinal pain**.
Not for cramps or backache mild—
But **neuro causes** reconciled.
Side effects? A sleepy crew:
Drowsiness, dry mouth, BP too.
Hypotension, dizziness, weak legs,
And sometimes liver issues beg.
So **monitor**: LFTs in range,
And **BP** for a sudden change.
Watch out for **fatigue** so deep,
They nap through life, not just sleep.
Teach patients: don't rise too quick—
That **orthostatic drop** is slick.
And don't drink booze while this is on—
It **doubles drowsy** before long.
Taper slowly if you stop—
Or **rebound hypertension** may pop.
And take with food if GI's stirred,
To smooth the ride and soothe the nerve.

No black box warning, but with care—
Because **sedation** waits out there.
And driving? Best delay the ride
Until alertness can decide.
Drug interactions? Yes, a few:
CYP1A2 comes into view.
Fluvoxamine and **ciprofloxacin**
Can spike the levels—heart may spin.
So **Zanaflex**, though small and still,
Can **loosen spastic muscles** at will.
With care and timing, dose by dose,
It helps the body move more close.

PYRIDOSTIGMINE (MESTINON)

Acetylcholinesterase Inhibitor / Myasthenia Gravis Agent

When **muscles tire** before their time,
And **simple tasks** feel like a climb,
Pyridostigmine lends a hand—
To help the nerves and muscles stand.
It **blocks acetylcholinesterase**,
So **ACh** has **longer stays**.
This lets the signals cross the gap,
So movement flows without a snap.
Used in **myasthenia gravis** true,
Where strength is fleeting, weak, and few.
It boosts the **neuromuscular spark**,
So patients move from dim to bright.
Side effects? A cholinergic tide:
Sweating, **cramping**, tears may slide.
Diarrhea, bradycardia, too—
And **salivation** might come through.
If **overdosed**, the symptoms show
A **cholinergic crisis** starts to grow:
Muscle twitching, respiratory low,
Can mimic worsening symptoms, though.
Monitor: muscle strength and tone,
And **respiratory function** all alone.
Adjust the dose to match their need—
Too much or little won't succeed.
Teach patients: space doses right,
To **time around their activity height**.
It kicks in fast, so plan ahead
Before they get out of bed.

No black box warning, still stay wise
To signs of **overdose in disguise**.
Differentiate the **crisis state**—
Myasthenic vs. cholinergic fate.
Drug interactions? Yes, a few—
With **atropine**, it can undo.
And be aware of meds that block
The **neuromuscular junction's talk**.
So **Mestinon**, with purpose clear,
Helps bring lost strength a bit more near.
With careful timing, dose, and plan,
It helps the weak to stand again.

SCOPOLAMINE PATCH (TRANSDERM SCOP)
Anticholinergic - Motion Sickness & Nausea Prevention

When nausea strikes before the trip, And spinning seas begin to grip, The **Scopolamine patch** steps in, To settle motion deep within.

It's an **anticholinergic**, smooth and sly, That blocks **muscarinic** nerves nearby. By halting **acetylcholine's sway**, It keeps the brain's reflex at bay.

Used for **motion sickness dread**, Like boats and cars and spinning head. Also in **post-op** nausea, too— To calm the waves when meds feel new.

The patch goes **behind the ear**, real neat, And works for **three days** on repeat. Apply it **four hours** in advance, So your balance stands a fighting chance.

It's **transdermal**, slow and sure, A steady dose to help endure. Absorbs through skin into the stream, So you don't lose it if you scream.

Side effects are mostly dry: **Dry mouth**, **blurry vision**, eye. **Drowsiness**, or **dizzy tilt**, And **urinary retention** guilt.

It may cause **confusion**, more in age, So caution in that patient stage. Elder folks may lose their grip, Or fall because of one small strip.

Remove it once the trip is done, Then wash your hands—don't touch for fun. If it gets into **eyes**, beware— **Dilated pupils** may be there.

It interacts with **other drying meds**, Like **antihistamines** or sleepy heads. So check for burden on the brain, Before applying it again.

Not for kids below the line Of **sixteen years**, unless assigned. And in **pregnancy**, assess the weight— It's **Category C**, so moderate.

So for motion, cruise, or post-op drop, You'll reach for **Transderm Scop** nonstop. One little patch, a tidy friend— To make the world stop spin and bend.

TOVIAZ (FESOTERODINE)

Anticholinergic - Neurogenic Bladder & Overactive Bladder

When bladder nerves have lost their way, And leaks or urges rule the day, **Toviaz**, or **Fesoterodine**, Can help restore a calm routine.

It's an **anticholinergic** med, That quiets what the bladder said. By blocking **M3 receptors** tight, It slows those spasms out of sight.

It treats the **neurogenic type**, Where spinal signals aren't quite right. Also helps with **OAB**, Where urgency won't go away.

The med relaxes **detrusor muscle**, So urine flows without the hustle. And increases the bladder's hold, So sudden loss can be controlled.

It comes in **extended-release** form, Once daily dose becomes the norm. No crushing, breaking, or split plan— Just swallow whole per doctor's scan.

Side effects that may appear: **Dry mouth**, **constipation**, maybe smear. **Blurred vision**, **drowsy**, **headache**, too— The usual anticholinergic crew.

Use caution in the **elderly**, As **falls** and **confusion** risk may be. And never mix with drugs that slow The bladder, bowels, or pressure flow.

Avoid in **narrow-angle glaucoma**, And in **urinary retention trauma**. Also screen for **GI blocks**, To prevent some major shocks.

It's processed in the **liver space**, So **hepatic issues** slow the pace. Use **CYP3A4** knowledge wise— Strong inhibitors raise the highs.

It's not a cure, but symptom balm, To help the bladder stay more calm. When **neurogenic** roots disrupt, This med can help folks hold things up.

So if the bladder can't comply, And leaks or urges multiply, Try **Toviaz**, a daily guide— To help the nerves and flow collide.

Part X
Miscellaneous Neurology

ACETAZOLAMIDE (DIAMOX)
Carbonic Anhydrase Inhibitor

A **carbonic anhydrase inhibitor** it be,
It blocks the enzyme, quite cleverly.
Stops reabsorption of **bicarb and salt**,
So fluid drops—and pressure halts.
Used for **glaucoma** and **altitude woes**,
Seizures, **edema**—the list just grows.
It **lowers ICP** in neuroland,
Reducing pressure, just as planned.

Side effects can bring some strife:
Tingling, nausea, altered life.
Kidney stones, fatigue, and taste,
Metabolic acidosis—no time to waste.
Check labs for electrolytes that shift,
Bicarb, potassium—they may drift.
Watch for signs the **CNS is blue**,
Like **confusion** or a **mental skew**.

Tell patients: **take it with some food**,
It might upset if taken nude.
Warn them of the **pee increase**,
And **sulfa allergies**—watch for these!
There's a **black box**? No, not here,
But still, stay cautious, stay sincere.
Avoid with **high-dose aspirin**, too,
It alters how the drug gets through.

So **Acetazolamide** makes fluid flee,
Relieves the pressure gracefully.
With proper care and patient talk,
This med can help their neurons walk.

AMIFAMPRIDINE (FIRDAPSE)
Potassium Channel Blocker

For muscles weak that tire fast,
Amifampridine helps them last.
It **blocks K⁺ channels** to extend,
The **ACh signal** at the end.
It boosts the nerve's electric beat,
So **muscle fibers** can repeat.
Used for **Lambert-Eaton Myasthenic** plight,
Where **strength returns** with every bite.

Side effects you need to flag:
Seizures, most serious—watch that tag.
Also **paresthesia**, tingles creep,
And **GI upset** may not sleep.
Abdominal pain, and **nausea, too**,
Plus **insomnia** that won't undo.
Back pain, **dizziness**, blurred-out sight—
So monitor them day and night.

Nursing considerations include:
Start low and go slow with this dude.
Avoid if there's a **seizure past**,
And renal caution—**dose won't last**.
Check renal function before the ride,
And if there's **hepatic disease**, best to hide.
No food with dose? Nah, that's fine,
Just space them out on **schedule time**.

Teach patients not to **double take**,
If they miss one—**no big mistake**.
But seizures? That's a **911** cue—
Stop the drug and follow through.
No **black box**, but **seizure risk** is real,
Especially with meds that seal
That risk, like **bupropion** or the line
Of **CNS stimulants**—decline.

So **Firdapse** brings the signal back,
To nerves that faded off the track.
With proper care, it lights the spark,
And helps weak muscles make their mark.

CANNABIDIOL (EPIDIOLEX)

Anticonvulsant / Cannabinoid (CBD)

From **cannabis**, but won't get you high,
Cannabidiol helps seizures fly.
It's pure **CBD**, not THC,
And **Epidiolex** sets symptoms free.
It's approved for **rare seizure storms**,
Like **Lennox-Gastaut** and **Dravet forms**.
Also helps with **TSC** (tuberous strain),
To calm the brain from constant pain.

It works through **mechanisms unknown**,
Though **calcium channels** might be shown.
And **GPR55** may play a part—
It slows the storm and soothes the heart.
Side effects can sometimes land:
Drowsiness, diarrhea, low appetite hand.
Liver enzyme rises—a must to track,
And **infections** may sneak in the back.

Monitor with labs on file:
LFTs at baseline, then each while.
Especially with **valproate**, take care,
That combo gives **liver risks** to spare.
Teach patients to **dose with food**—
It helps the **absorption** and the mood.
Tell them not to **mix with booze**,
And report if they feel confused.

No **black box warning**, but stay sharp—
Suicidal thoughts may leave a mark.
So screen for mood and mental state,
And intervene if things aren't great.
Drug interactions? Oh yes—prepare:
It's metabolized through **CYP3A4's** lair.
Watch **clobazam, valproate**, and more,
As levels shift or side effects soar.

So **Epidiolex**, smooth and clean,
Brings calm where chaos once had been.
A plant-born gift, with science flair,
That helps the brain breathe clearer air.

DALFAMPRIDINE (AMPYRA)

Potassium Channel Blocker / MS Agent

When **MS** slows the body's stride,
And walking strength begins to slide,
Dalfampridine lends some fire,
To help those **weakened limbs aspire**.
It **blocks potassium channels** tight,
To **prolong nerve signals** day and night.
It helps the neurons fire with grace,
So legs can find a **steadier pace**.

Approved for **walking in MS alone**,
But not for types with tremors shown.
It's not a cure, but helps restore
The **speed and stride** some had before.
Side effects to watch with care:
UTIs, insomnia, dizziness flare.
Headache, nausea, and some may find
Seizures lurking close behind.

Yes—**seizure risk** is key to note,
Especially if **dose floats the wrong boat**.
Never **double up** if one is missed—
That's how seizures join the list.
Monitor kidney function, too,
Creatinine clearance under 50?
Then no can do.
It's **renally cleared**, so dose must match
Or adverse effects may soon dispatch.

Teach patients: **take 12 hours apart**,
Don't crush, chew, or break the part.
No more than **two a day**, that's it—
Overdose can bring a seizure hit.
No **black box**, but still be wise—
The seizure risk is no disguise.
And **interactions**? Not a ton,
But avoid **compounding seizure fun**.

So **Ampyra**, while it won't erase,
The root of MS's slowing pace,
Can help improve the way folks walk—
With steady steps and careful talk.

DEUTETRABENAZINE (AUSTEDO)

VMAT2 Inhibitor / Tardive Dyskinesia & Chorea Agent

When **involuntary movements** won't quit,
And limbs or face just won't sit,
Deutetrabenazine joins the fight,
To help bring twitching back to right.
It's a **VMAT2 inhibitor** clean,
That blocks **dopamine in the machine**.
By limiting what neurons store,
It calms the shakes and flails and more.
Used for **Huntington's chorea pain**,
And **tardive dyskinesia** in the brain.
It smooths out **jerky, sudden flow**,
To help the body **move with control**.
But like all drugs, side effects stay:
Sedation, dry mouth, mood decay.
Diarrhea, fatigue, and sometimes low
Appetite may come or go.
Most serious? **Suicidal thought**,
Especially if depression's already fought.
So screen for **mood disorders** true,
And watch how symptoms rise or skew.
Monitor mood and mental state,
And check for **fall risk**—don't be late.
Start **twice a day**, with food preferred,
To lessen nausea that's incurred
Teach patients not to miss their med,
And don't stop suddenly—stepwise instead.
No alcohol or sedative play,
Or motor control might drift away.
Black box warning? Yes—be wise:
Depression and **suicide** may rise.
Especially in **Huntington's disease**,
Where psychiatric risks are not at ease
Drug interactions? Some are key:
MAOIs? No—serotonin storm could be.
Caution with **CYP2D6 inhibitors** near—
Like **fluoxetine, paroxetine**—stay clear.
So **Austedo**, though not well-known,
Gives **movement disorders** a calmer tone.
It works with grace when others stall—
But needs close watch through it all.

DEXTROMETHORPHAN/ QUINIDINE (NUEDEXTA)

NMDA Receptor Antagonist + CYP2D6 Inhibitor / Pseudobulbar Affect Agent

When **tears or laughter** break through wrong,
And **emotions feel too loud or long**,
Nuedexta steps in to realign,
The signals crossing over the line.
It's made of two unique components paired:
Dextromethorphan, finely prepared—
An **NMDA blocker** in disguise,
That **modulates glutamate** highs.
And **Quinidine**? A smaller dose—
Just enough to help **DM last most**.
It **inhibits CYP2D6**, you see,
So **dextro** sticks around effectively.
Used to treat **Pseudobulbar Affect's tide**,
When **laughs or sobs** can't be denied.
In **ALS**, **MS**, and stroke, it's shown
To help those **involuntary tones**.
Side effects may soon arise:
Dizziness, **diarrhea**, and **falls** surprise.
Swelling, **cough**, and sometimes **QT prolong**,
So cardiac risk must be **ruled out strong**.
Monitor ECG in those with past **Heart issues**, or if **QT's too vast**.
Also check **drug levels** that rely
On **CYP2D6**—they may amplify.
Teach patients this won't **change the mood**,
But it can **help the tears subdued**.
Tell them to **take with food or not**,
But **missed doses**? Skip—don't double the shot.
No **black box warning** here to share,
But still, approach with extra care.
Especially if **heart failure** is near,
Or **arrhythmias** ever appear.
Drug interactions? Yes, a few:
Avoid with **MAOIs** or **flu**-crew.
Serotonin syndrome risk may rise,
With **SSRIs**, **tramadol**, **linezolid** ties.
So **Nuedexta**, though a bit obscure,
Can help where PBA feels unsure.
It reins in tears or out-of-place cheer,
And offers control when none feels near.

DROXIDOPA (NORTHERA)
Alpha/Beta Agonist Prodrug / Neurogenic Orthostatic Hypotension Agent

When **standing up** brings **dizzy spins**,
And blood flow loss begins and wins,
Droxidopa lends a lift,
To **raise the pressure**, smooth and swift.
It's a **prodrug** turned to **norepinephrine**,
Boosting signals the nerves aren't givin'.
It **stimulates alpha and beta** flow,
To help the **BP rise—not go**.
Used for **neurogenic low BP**,
Like in **Parkinson's** or **MSD**.
When nerves can't signal vessels tight,
Northera helps them hold upright
Side effects? A few to share:
Headache, nausea, hypertension scare.
Fatigue, dizziness, and **chest pain**,
Falls, UTIs, or **tingling brain**.
Supine hypertension is the risk—
So lying down can turn quite brisk.
BP at night must be observed,
To keep that balance finely curved.
Monitor BP while lying flat,
And upright too—imagine that!
Check for **cardiac signs or strain**,
And watch for pressure that won't wane.
Teach patients: **don't take late at night**,
To prevent BP rising out of sight.
And if they feel a pounding chest,
Pause the med and call for test.
No black box warning here today,
But still, the **BP rise** can sway.
Especially in **elderly hearts**,
Start low and slow with thoughtful charts.
Drug interactions? Sure, a few—
With **MAOIs**, say a bold adieu.
Caution with other **pressors** tight,
That might cause BP spikes overnight.
So **Droxidopa**, niche but key,
Gives upright folks some stability.
With careful dose and eyes on track,
It helps the BP **bounce right back**.

EDARAVONE (RADICAVA)
Free Radical Scavenger / ALS Agent

When **neurons fail** and muscles fade,
And **ALS** brings its silent cascade,
Edaravone steps in the stream,
To fight the **oxidative dream**.
A **free radical scavenger** true,
It helps protect what nerves still do.
Though it won't reverse or cure the slide,
It may help **slow the weakening tide**.
It's used for **ALS**, that hard decline,
To preserve the **function left in line**.
It quiets the damage done by stress,
From **oxidants** in excess.
Side effects are often few,
But here are some to look into:
Bruising, gait issues, headache pain,
Skin inflammation, confusion strain.
More serious but rare?
Hypersensitivity,
Anaphylaxis lacks amenity.
Especially with **sulfite ties**,
So check those allergies before it flies.
Monitor for signs of rash or breath,
Especially during the **infusion depth**.
Also watch for **gait decline**,
To track disease and dosing line.
Teach patients it comes **IV**,
Given in cycles—**10 or 14 days**, then free.

There's also an **oral form** to use,
With timing and food-checks to peruse.
No black box warning, but stay alert—
For signs of allergy that can hurt.
Sodium bisulfite may trigger scare,
So avoid in those who can't go there.
Drug interactions? Nothing strong,
It doesn't ride the CYP line long.
But always check with **other meds**,
Especially those with **neuro threads**.
So **Edaravone**, subtle and kind,
Shields the neurons left behind.
A quiet hero in ALS's war,
Protecting cells just a little more.

LIDOCAINE PATCH (LIDODERM)
Local Anesthetic / Sodium Channel Blocker

When **nerves ignite** in skin and bone,
And **burning pain** won't leave you alone,
Lidocaine patches calm the flame—
A **topical fix** for **nerve pain's name**.
It **blocks sodium channels** at the gate,
To stop pain signals from reaching late.
No full numbness, just relief,
From **postherpetic neuralgia grief**.
Used for **localized nerve-type pain**,
Applied to skin to **ease the strain**.
It's not for burns or wounds that seep—
Just **intact skin**, shallow and deep.
Side effects? They're mostly mild:
Redness, itching, burning styled.
But in rare systemic case,
It may cause **CNS distress**.
Monitor if too many are worn—
Or if they're cut, or skin is torn.
Too much absorbed could bring a scare:
Tremors, confusion, even **air hunger** there.
Teach patients: wear it **12 hours on**,
Then **12 hours off**—that's how it's drawn.
Don't use heat or wrap it tight,
Or too much drug could take a flight.
Also don't **cut** it unless told—
That changes how the drug unfolds.
Wash hands after, keep it flat,
And stick to limits—**no more than 3 patches** at.
No black box warning, but stay alert,
Especially if the heart's been hurt.
Large doses near the **chest or spine**
Could cross into conduction line.
Drug interactions? Not too many—
But if combined with other **anesthetics**—any
IV or topical dose nearby
May raise the risk of levels high.
So **Lidoderm**, with surface grace,
Brings comfort to that burning place.
A patch of calm for nerve-stung skin,
To help the healing work begin.

RILUZOLE (RILUTEK)
Glutamate Inhibitor / ALS Disease-Modifying Agent

When **muscles weaken**, breath grows tight,
And **ALS** steals day from night,
Riluzole gives time some grace—
To slow the loss, not win the race.
It's not a cure, but **buys more days**,
By working through **glutamate's wild blaze**.
It blocks release and cuts the tide
Of signals that cause motor cells to slide.

Used in **amyotrophic lateral sclerosis**,
To **extend survival**, though the gain is modest.
It helps delay **ventilator time**,
And gives some **function** back its climb.
Side effects? A few to name:
Nausea, dizziness, fatigue in frame.
Liver enzymes may rise with use,
So **LFT monitoring** is a must—no excuse.

Monitor: ALT, AST,
Every month, then quarterly.
If values soar beyond the mark,
It's time to hold or disembark.
Teach patients: take it **on an empty belly**,
1 hour before food—or after, not smelly.
Twice a day is how it's done,
With water, not with food or fun.

No black box warning, but be aware
Of signs like **jaundice**, which aren't rare.
And though it's safe in many crowds,
It's not for those with liver shrouds.
Drug interactions? CYPs apply—
CYP1A2 is the main guy.
So **smoking** may reduce the med,
While **Cipro** raises it instead.

So **Riluzole**, the quiet guide,
Stands by the ALS patient's side.
Not a cure, but a steady hand,
To help them walk a bit more land.

RISDIPLAM (EVRYSDI)

SMN2 Splicing Modifier / Spinal Muscular Atrophy (SMA) Therapy

When **muscles fade** before their time,
And tiny bodies cannot climb,
Risdiplam steps in with care—
To help the gene express what's fair.
It's a **splicing modifier**, new and wise,
For **SMN2**, it changes ties.
So more **SMN protein** flows,
And muscle strength more slowly goes.

Used for **SMA types 1 through 3**,
In infants, kids, and adults you see.
It's an **oral liquid** once a day—
No injections in the fray.
Side effects? A gentle list:
Fever, rash, and **GI twist.**
Mouth ulcers, **joint pain**, **runny nose**,
And sometimes **urinary tract woes**.

Monitor: liver labs and weight,
And **eye development**—don't wait.
Pulmonary function, where needed, too,
In older patients pulling through.
Teach caregivers how to pour:
It's based on weight—and **no food before**
Or after—at least **30 minutes** clear,
So the drug absorbs without a smear.

No black box warning, but still wise
To track for signs as strength may rise.
It's **not a cure**, but slows decline,
So children hold more life in line.
Drug interactions? Not a lot—
But **CYP enzymes** still have a spot.
So watch with meds that share that track,
And **renal or hepatic** setbacks.

So **Evrysdi**, a liquid beam,
Brings hope to families who dream.
With daily dose and genes in play,
It helps keep strength from fading away.

SODIUM OXYBATE (XYREM)

CNS Depressant / GABA-B Agonist / Narcolepsy Agent

When **sleep attacks** hit like a wave,
And **cataplexy** steals what you gave,
Sodium Oxybate calms the spin—
To bring **real sleep** back deep within.
It's a form of **GHB**, you see,
But used in sleep **therapeutically**.
It binds to **GABA-B**, smooth and low,
To help **slow-wave cycles** start to grow.
Used in **narcolepsy** at night,
To reduce **cataplexy** and make days bright.
It helps with **daytime sleep attacks**,
By giving nighttime sleep more tracks.
Side effects? You must take care:
Nausea, confusion, breathing rare.
Sleepwalking, bedwetting, dizzy light,
And next-day fog from sleep too tight.
Black box warning? Absolutely yes—
It's **CNS depression**, serious stress.
Abuse, misuse, and **respiratory fall**,
Especially with **alcohol** in the hall.
It's **Schedule III**, but **Xywav's** near—
A **low-sodium** version some prefer clear.
Still tightly controlled, and rightly so—
Because of **GHB's** street-level glow.
Monitor: **mood, breathing**, and their tone,
Especially if they sleep alone.
And track for **falls, mental decline**,
Or signs that they're not taking fine.
Teach patients: take it **in two doses**,
One at bedtime, the other **mid-slumber's closest**.
On an **empty stomach**, that's the key,
Or absorption's lost to chemistry.
Drug interactions? Avoid the stack
Of **CNS depressants**—pull them back.
No **alcohol, benzos**, or deep sedatives,
Unless you like ER narratives.
So **Xyrem**, powerful, short, and deep,
Helps **narcoleptics** finally sleep.
But only used with strict control,
To keep both **benefit** and **safety whole**.

TETRABENAZINE (XENAZINE)

VMAT2 Inhibitor / Huntington's Chorea & Tardive Dyskinesia Agent

When **movements twist** beyond control,
And **chorea robs** the body's role,
Tetrabenazine steps in tight—
To **dull the dance** and calm the fight.
It **blocks VMAT2**, no delay,
So **dopamine** is tucked away.
With less to flood the basal crew,
Those jerky motions may subdue.
Used in **Huntington's disease** most known,
Where limbs and face have minds their own.
And sometimes used for **tardive twitch**,
Though **off-label** guides that niche.
Side effects? They must be weighed:
Depression, **suicidal shade**.
Sedation, **fatigue**, and **dizzy light**,
And **parkinsonism** may take a bite.
So **black box warning**? Yes, it's there—
For **suicide risk**, so **mental care**.
Especially in those who've had the dark,
This med should come with extra spark.
Monitor: mood, and energy,
Sleep, **balance**, and activity.
EKG for QT's stretch,
And **neuro checks** you'll often fetch.
Teach patients: take it with a meal,
And **titrate slow** to see how they feel.

Three times daily is the plan,
But dosing varies by each hand.
Drug interactions? Yes—some real:
Avoid with **MAOIs**, that's the deal.
And with **reserpine**, wait a while,
Or side effects will stack and pile.
Also, **CYP2D6** has a role—
So if they're a **poor metabolizer**, control
The dose with care, or choose anew,
And watch for levels rising through.
So **Xenazine**, precise and rare,
Helps ease the moves that aren't fair.
But always used with thoughtful guide—
With mood and safety side by side.

VALBENAZINE (INGREZZA)
VMAT2 Inhibitor / Tardive Dyskinesia Agent

When **tardive tics** won't slow or fade,
From meds that antipsychs have made,
Valbenazine steps in the stream—
To soften movements that **shouldn't be seen**.
It **inhibits VMAT2** with care,
So **dopamine's transport** is less in the air.
That means less flood in movement zones,
And fewer **grimaces**, **twists**, or **groans**.

Used for **tardive dyskinesia's grace**,
From antipsychs that **shift the face**.
It helps restore control and tone,
So patients feel more **like their own**.
Side effects? The list is small:
Sleepiness, and sometimes a **fall**.
Fatigue, **QT prolongation** slight,
So **EKGs** may guide the light.

Monitor: heart rhythm and gait,
Especially if **cardiac history** waits.
And check for **sedation**, mood, or drift,
To make sure balance doesn't shift.
Teach patients: one pill a day,
With or without food, either way.
It works best with **consistent use**,
And should not be a med to lose.

No black box warning, but stay sharp—
Especially if they **drive or harp**
On feeling tired, slowed, or hazed—
Adjust the dose if they seem dazed.
Drug interactions? Yes, beware—
CYP3A4 is active there.
Inhibitors like **clarithromycin**
May raise levels—adjust within.

So **Ingrezza**, with modern stride,
Helps tame the movements one can't hide.
A once-a-day, well-tolerated ride—
To bring back peace from the inside.

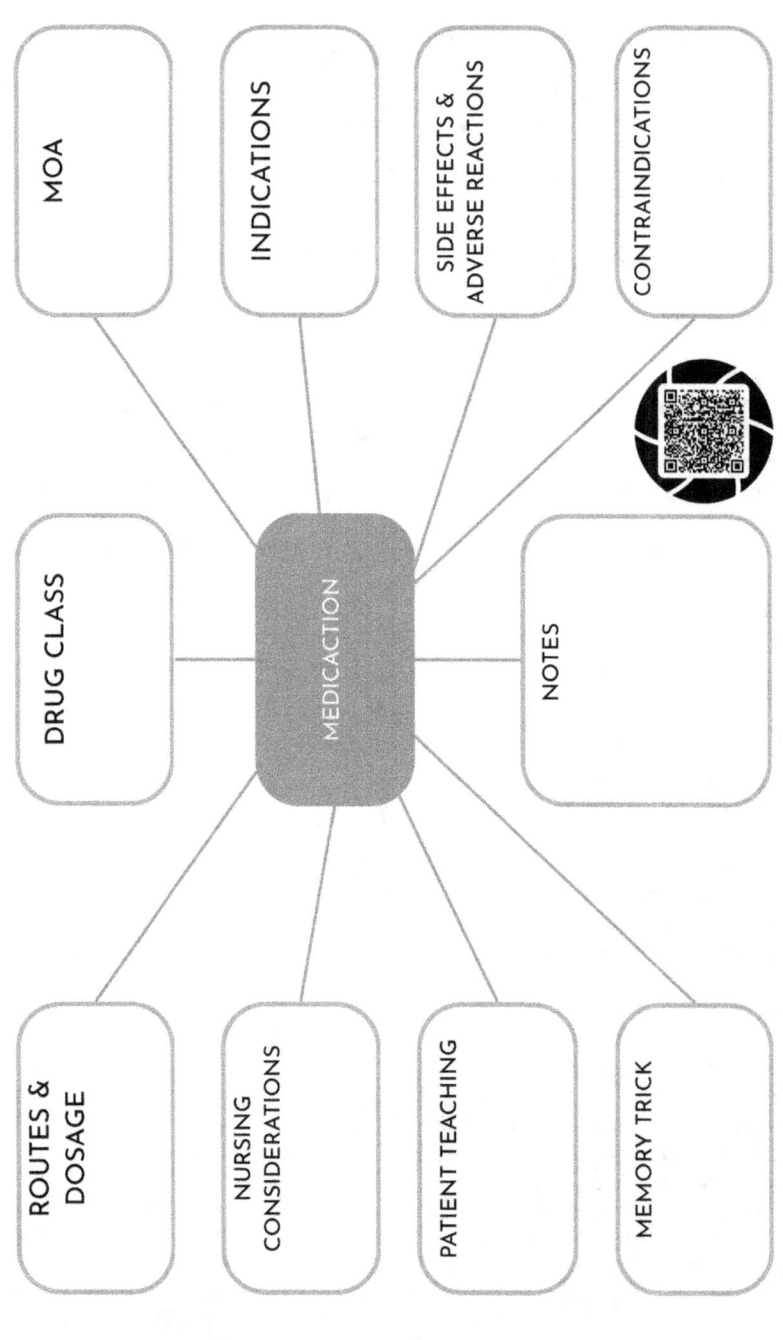

THANK YOU

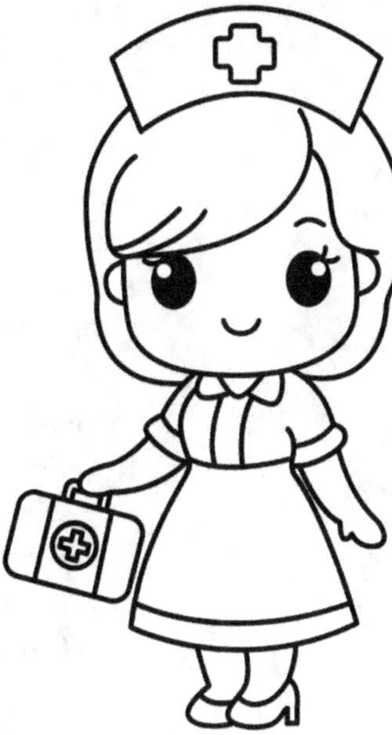

for getting this book and for making it all the way to the end!

Before you go, I wanted to ask you for one small favor. Could you please consider posting a review? Because posting a review is the best and easiest way to support the work of independent authors like me.

Your feedback will help me a ton!

Click **Here** or Scan the QR code below!

OTHER TITLES IN THE MADE EASY SERIES

Geriatrics Made Easy
Emergency Care Made Easy
Critical Care Made Easy
Human Growth & Development
Maternal & Newborn Made Easy
Mental Health Made Easy
Organic Chemistry Made Easy
General Chemistry Made Easy
Pediatrics Made Easy
Med-Surg Made Easy, Vol 1
Med-Surg Made Easy, Vol 2
Microbiology Made Easy
Nursing Skills & Procedures
Pathophysiology Made Easy
Nursing Assessment Made Easy
Nutrition Made Easy
Anatomy & Physiology Vol 1
Anatomy & Physiology Vol 2

Pharmacology Series

Pharmacology Made Easy Vol 1
Pharmacology Made Easy Vol 2
Pharmacology Made Easy Vol 3
Oncology Meds Made Easy
Cardiac Meds Made Easy
Endocrine Meds Made Easy
Pain Meds Made Easy
GI Meds Made Easy
Respiratory Meds Made Easy
Critical Meds Made Easy
ER/ICU Meds Made Easy
Neuro Meds Made Easy
Psych Meds Made Easy
Pediatric Meds Made Easy
OB/GYN Meds Made Easy

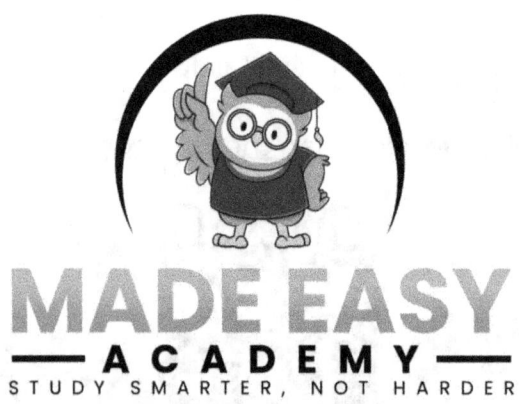